WE ARE ALL LIVING WITH HIV

WE ARE ALL LIVING WITH HIV

HOW TO SET POLICIES AND GUIDELINES FOR THE WORKPLACE

Earl C. Pike and Phil Greasley

FREE ASSOCIATION BOOKS / LONDON

Published in 1997 by
Free Association Books Ltd
57 Warren Street, London W1P 5PA

US edition first published in 1993 by Deaconess Press

ISBN 1 85343 372 1

A CIP catalogue record for this book is available from the British Library.

Produced for Free Association Books by
Chase Production Services, Chadlington, OX7 3LN
Printed in the EC by J.W. Arrowsmith Ltd, Bristol

Contents

Preface

A Note from the UK Author about the Original USA Book

This book was first published in the USA in 1993. Earl C. Pike was the sole author and the original title was *We are All Living with AIDS: How you can set Policies and Guidelines for the Workplace.*

My aim was to adapt the book to make it relevant and accessible to the UK. Originally, achieving this aim seemed only a matter of re-writing chapters dealing with employment law, testing and confidentiality. The end result, however, is that the book has been considerably modified throughout. The chapters with the least changes are Chapters 7 and 8 although modifications have been made in these to make the concepts and language applicable to the UK.

The UK version is also considerably shorter than the American version. This is because I have tried not to duplicate information which is already available in the UK. For example, I have not included sections on the clinical care of people with HIV because I believe that the NHS, the associated unions and the independent sector have already provided excellent models in this area. I also decided not to include guidelines and sample policies for specific organisations, such as those dealing with homelessness and drug use. Again, information is already available about many specialist areas. 'Useful Information and Addresses' given in Appendix 3 gives some pointers about where other information can be found.

Despite the changes made to the book, the essence remains the same. There is the same approach to policy, the same messages expressed and the same commitment to opposing discrimination against people with HIV and

AIDS. As an endorsement to this, a section from Earl's introduction is reproduced below:

> I wanted to write *We are All Living with AIDS* because I was frustrated, and because I suspect that you may be frustrated as well.
>
> We are now in the second decade of the HIV/AIDS epidemic. Friends of mine have died from this disease, and I will probably see more people, people I love, die before the whole thing is over. You, the reader, may have had the same experience.
>
> For far too long far too little was done to recognize, face and address HIV and its effects on millions of people. Many individuals – and agencies and businesses and governments – were too frightened, too appalled, too angry, too repulsed, too occupied, too whatever to respond. Even some of the best-intentioned people were sometimes hoping that the whole terrifying, confusing disease would just go away. It didn't, and it won't anytime soon.
>
> And consulting with workplaces of almost every stripe, serving a wide variety of clients and customers, I have come to recognize how critical the organization's role is, and will be, in fighting this epidemic – both in terms of treating clients and employees with HIV or AIDS well, and in terms of providing education and support for behavior change to reduce the transmission of HIV.

The Red Ribbon

The origins of the red ribbon (depicted on the cover of this book) as a symbol for concern about HIV and AIDS are vague, but it is commonly believed to be a creation of the USA group 'Visual AIDS' which introduced it in 1991.

Wearing a red ribbon has become popular, even somewhat trendy in a few circles. Some AIDS activists even contend that it has lost its meaning through overuse. Others still consider the ribbon a source of both financial assistance (since it is sometimes used to raise funds) and moral support for people living with HIV or AIDS.

Wear the ribbon. As a symbol, it's important. But remember: it should never be a hollow gesture. Wear it as a commitment to do something about HIV and AIDS, as a promise to remember, as a dedication to work for an end to discrimination, an end to isolation and rejection, an end to hate. Wear it; make it mean something.

Dedication and Acknowledgements to the US Edition

Dedication

It is perhaps uncustomary to provide a dedication for a book of this kind. But the fight against HIV and AIDS has challenged, and rightfully so, much that is 'customary', and one more challenge cannot hurt. I therefore dedicate this book to Perry Tilleraas, Eric Lerner and 'Wee-zee' Hoeschler, whose passions and loves in the fight against AIDS helped many of us remember what it was all about: that our lives are tempestuous, sometimes heavy with pain and sometimes wild with joy, and ultimately, always, precious and sacred.

Acknowledgements

There are at least three groups of people I need to acknowledge for their generous assistance and support in the development of this book.

First of all, I want to thank the Minnesota AIDS Funding Consortium and my project liaison, Mary Hunter. They provided me with a grant that gave me the time, freedom and economic resources to write the book, and were patient with my requests for help (and extensions of deadlines).

When I first started on *We are All Living with AIDS*, I realised that it would be a good idea to assemble a sort of personal advisory committee – a group that could guide me and perhaps, as needed, tell me I was off-base. I gathered together a small team of people whose thinking about HIV and related issues I trusted a great deal, who I respected personally, politically and intellectually. They were fantastic.

The committee was composed of the following people, the second group to which I owe my heartfelt appreciation:

Jolynn Blaeser, Leo Guzman, Elizabeth Klein, Jennifer Reinhart, Stella West, Sharon Day, Jonathan Hanft, Fraser Nelson, Sally Swallen, Cindy Zegers, Janet Flood, Mary Hunter, Tim Reardon, Kim Sundet.

And the following people reviewed various drafts of the book, and provided incisive feedback and advice. Their comments and viewpoints were invaluable (organisational affiliations are listed for purposes of identification only).

Cordelia Anderson, Sensibilities, Inc.
Julia Ashley, Minnesota AIDS Project
Terry Backhaus, West Central Community Service Center (Willmar, MN)
Sara Baron, St Paul Red Cross
Lori Beaulieu, Minnesota Indian Women's Resource Center
Linda Brandt, Rural AIDS Action Network
Dan Capouch, Hennepin County (MN) Social Services
Kevin Cwayna MD, Hemophilia Treatment Center
Lori Dablow, Developmental Disabilities Division, MN Dept of Human Services
Norma Denbrook, Corrections AIDS Prevention Program, Hennepin County (MN) Community Health
Nancy Devitt, Hennepin County (MN) Planning
Cayle Dixon, Minnesota AIDS Project Legal Program
Vern Drilling, LaMancha Corporation
Linda Ernst, Minneapolis Red Cross
Dorothy Flynn, Hazelden Institute
Tom Flynn, private consultant
Dan Ford, Minnesota AIDS Project
Karen Helfand, Chicanos Latinos Unidos en Servicios
Carlton Hogan, Community Programs for Clinical Research on AIDS (Statistical Centers)
Mariann Johnson, Arts Over AIDS
Sara Judson, private consultant
Kara Korach, St Paul Jewish Community Center
Pat Lamb, Employee Assistance Program, Cargill Corporation

Frank Lamendola, Journeywell
Susan Langston, Hennepin County (MN) Social Services
Al Mayotte, Austin Community College
Beth O'Neill, Chicago AIDS Foundation
Carolyn Patierno, Sex Education and Information Council of the US (New York)
Barb Perrin, Abbott Northwestern Chemical Dependency Treatment Program
Frank Rhame MD, University of Minnesota Hospitals
Jim Rothenberger, University of Minnesota School of Public Health
Steven Schaefer, Ramsey Hospital HIV Program
Sandra Schwartzer, New Beginnings at Waverly
Tom Soles, Crisis Connection
Patsy Stinchfield, Children's Hospital
Scott Strickland MD, Park-Nicollet Medical Center
Edward Wedman, Deaconess Press, Fairview Hospital and Healthcare Services
Taylor Wilcox, Youth and AIDS Program

For their assistance and support, thanks also go to: Mike Moen, Minnesota Department of Health; Ruth Ellen Luehr, Minnesota Department of Education; and Carol Falkowski, Minnesota Department of Human Services.

Finally, I would be remiss if I failed to extend my ongoing thanks to Jay Johnson, my editor at Deaconess Press, whose unfailing commitment to this project (as well as some appropriate nagging) helped shepherd its completion.

And, as always, my immeasurable thanks to EDK.

Earl C. Pike

Acknowledgements to the UK Edition

Thanks to Simon Walsh at Immunity for suggesting to Free Association Books that I might be interested in writing/adapting the UK version of this book; to Carol Merchant for early work on the Disability Discrimination Act – a useful starting point for Chapter 3; thanks to Earl C. Pike for writing the USA version in the first place and to Free Association Books for publishing the UK version.

Thanks to all my friends and family for putting up with me saying 'No, I'm sorry I can't, I've got this book to finish.' Special thanks to my partner, Chris, for encouragement.

Phil Greasley

Introduction

Many workplaces still have not developed policies to incorporate HIV or provided education about HIV. It is not merely that workplaces have been resistant to dealing with HIV and related issues – though, certainly, HIV has evoked a lot of strong emotional reactions. Many organisations – or more accurately the people within them – have just not thought that the issue is of relevance to them. Many other workplaces have not developed policies because they do not know how and, sometimes, they do not even know where to start.

It is not for lack of intelligence or sophistication or, most of the time, caring. It is just that when you combine what seems like the complicated information about HIV with the range of feelings that usually attend the issue, it is no wonder that individuals and workplaces as a whole either ignore the issue or feel too overwhelmed to start.

If anything, organisations should be concerned about the absence of policy and the legal vulnerability that such absence creates. If your organisation does not have a policy, there is no reason to wait any longer; the epidemic is here, and the time is now.

This book does not try to convince you, the reader, that there is a need for HIV policy in the workplace. It is assumed that if you have picked up this book, it is because you already see that need. Rather, *We are All Living with HIV* is designed to help individuals and workplaces at every stage of policy development. The information in the book is also designed to give you the ammunition to argue why policies covering HIV should be adopted, improved or updated.

It is geared toward workplaces of every variety, and can be employed by directors, managers, personnel, line staff or trade unionists within those organisations. It discusses not only the specifics of HIV/AIDS policy, but also the particular and sometimes unique obstacles that individuals may encounter in the policy development process. It will help you and your organisation to prepare for HIV/AIDS.

The scope and layout of this book are designed so that you will find everything you need to develop policy and to be able to use it practically and effectively. The book can be read and used in many different ways. It is recommended, however, that before you start, you read the summaries of the chapters below to give you an idea of what you want to read first.

Before You Start

For some people this book will be useful for taking them through the whole process of learning about HIV and learning how to introduce the need for policy into an organisation. Other readers may already have considerable knowledge about HIV and/or policy development; in this case the reader may find the book more useful to back up the arguments they are using to persuade others in their organisation to adopt or improve their policies.

If you know very little about HIV you may well want to start at Chapter 1. However, some people who feel they know a lot about HIV may want to start reading at Chapter 8 and read earlier chapters as they seem to become relevant to the development of policy.

A brief summary of the chapters is as follows.

Chapter 1 gives a range of background information about HIV. The chapter gives a history of the virus; basic facts about HIV and the effects it can have; modes of transmission; risk reduction; health and safety procedures; HIV statistics and an introduction as to why HIV discrimination should be opposed.

For people who know little about HIV, it will give a broad introduction to the subject. For others it may be useful for helping to explain the need for policy in your organisation or to be used as training resources. The chapter is referred to several times in Chapter 8 for use at different stages of policy development.

Chapter 2 looks at employment law in the UK in relation to HIV. The chapter begins by describing the statutory employment laws which give rights to all employees regardless of their HIV status. It goes on to show how these laws relate to people who are HIV positive.

Chapter 3 explains how people who are HIV positive and symptomatic may be covered by the Disability Discrimination Act (DDA). The chapter explains the responsibilities that employers have, under Section 6 of the DDA, to make changes or modifications to the work environment for people with disabilities. The second half of the chapter gives detail about the specific adaptations and modifications that may be helpful for people with or recovering from HIV related illness.

Chapter 4 looks at the factors which employers should consider when addressing the issue of confidentiality in relation to HIV. The chapter starts by explaining the ethical and legal obligations to maintain confidential information about HIV, it goes on to give principles and policy points which can be adopted by all employers regardless of their size or type. The chapter goes on to discuss confidentiality issues which may only be relevant in certain types of organisation.

Chapter 5 explores some of the wider employment issues which arise in relation to the HIV antibody test. As with Chapter 4, it starts with general points applicable to all organisations. The chapter goes on to look at areas which are only relevant to some organisations.

Chapter 6 gives a range of examples of HIV related discrimination. It also discusses other forms of discrimination that people affected with HIV may experience because of their sexuality, sex or race. The second part of the chapter concentrates on lesbian and gay discrimination because the link between HIV and sexuality discrimination has been so acute.

Chapter 7 provides a comprehensive range of information, techniques and instruments which can be used to assess where the organisation is now and what needs to be done in relation to HIV. In this sense the chapter provides all the tools necessary to conduct an HIV audit. The chapter identifies different stages that an organisation may have reached in relation to HIV. Checklists and questionnaires are provided to assess what stage your organisation is at and what needs to be done to move forward.

Chapter 8 maps out all the stages involved in policy development and implementation from the very beginning to the end – from deciding the need for policy; researching facts about HIV and AIDS; surveying and assessing the organisation as it is now; planning and drafting the policy; through to implementation and evaluation.

Chapter 9 draws on material used in other parts of the book to provide suggestions for points or clauses which can be included in HIV/AIDS policies and policies addressing diversity: including policies on lesbians and gay men.

This chapter may be useful at several different stages of the development of policy described in Chapter 8. For example, it may be useful both early on in policy development, for ideas about the policy points which could be tailored to suit your own organisation and, later, as a checklist to ensure that all areas of major importance have been included within the organisation's policy.

Appendices show where ongoing and up-to-date information can be found in relation to HIV and employment and give information about how organisations can make a public commitment to opposing HIV discrimination.

The Ethical Basis for Policy

Before we begin to look at HIV policies, we should discuss the ethical foundations that support those policies. Those foundations are critical and should be brought out into the open, for they allow us to state clearly the values and beliefs that lead us to propagate HIV/AIDS policy in the first place.

The following ideas form the ethical basis for all that comes after:

☑ **Our goal is to affirm life and hope over death and despair. In the face of life-threatening illness, we want to help people live with HIV, not die from it.**

☑ **We need to respect the rights and dignity of all people. People with HIV deserve the same consideration and support as any other client or employee. And they may have a lot to teach us about ourselves, each other, and being alive.**

☑ **We need to affirm the individual's right to choose. A lot of choices face all of us in relation to HIV: strategies to reduce risk, whether or not to be tested, what medical treatment to choose, which doctor would be most effective, and so on. Everyone has the right to all the information they need to make a wise choice, and to make the choices that are uniquely appropriate for them.**

☑ **Our policies and procedures should be based on solid epidemiological and virological fact. Some of the information presented about HIV can seem confusing or contradictory, and sometimes the information is just plain inaccurate. In such cases we should search out the truth as the only basis for our actions.**

☑ **Our policies and strategies should be based on a positive view of human sexuality. Many people experience so much condemnation in relation to their sexuality that they are not likely to respond to further rejection. Despite different views about specific matters related to sexuality, most of us can agree that human sexuality itself is a positive force.**

☑ **Our policies and strategies should take a long-term perspective. Myopic views will no longer suffice; reliable indicators tell us that HIV is going to be around for a while. That indicates that we will need to develop policies and strategies that will last, not just something that will get us through the next few months.**

- ☑ **We need to recognise that the crisis of HIV/AIDS is not merely medical. Responding to HIV as only a medical crisis will neglect some of the most important features of the epidemic: sexuality and homophobia, drug use and how we feel about it, illness and death, and many others.**

- ☑ **We need to remember that HIV mainly tends to affect those who have already suffered oppression for other reasons. It is not just that people with HIV are mistreated because of their illness, they are just as often mistreated because they are, for example, gay and/or black and HIV infected. We need to take all of those realities into account and we should recognise and affirm the diversity of individuals and communities.**

- ☑ **We need to be careful not to 'blame the victim'. People with HIV have heard all too often, both overtly and subtly, that they are 'at fault' for their illness, that they are 'dirty', that they are 'sinners' or 'corrupt', and much more in a similar vein. Organisations cannot allow themselves to add to the negative messages people with HIV are already getting.**

- ☑ **We need to affirm the right of people with HIV to accurate information and good care. Practice and policy should aim for the best service that can be provided, rather than mere adequacy.**

- ☑ **And finally, if for whatever reason we cannot serve people with HIV fully, we have a responsibility to facilitate good service. If personal or organisational limitations prevent the provision of good service and information, we need to make sure that they can be accessed, even if it means, as it often will, that referrals have to be made.**

1 All the Basics for Education and Training

Introduction

The information in this chapter may be of use in several different ways. You may decide that overall you know very little about HIV and would like to start from the beginning to ensure what you do know is fact. The chapter tries to give a solid background to HIV and AIDS which should put the whole subject into perspective.

You may, however, feel you know a lot about HIV and have been given 'the facts and figures' a hundred times before. In this case, you may find the chapter more useful as a resource or source of reference. Most sections are written to stand alone as, for example, training and education materials or as background information for research or reports.[1] Equally there may be times when you are arguing for good policy or practice about HIV in your organisation and need to cross-check a few basic facts.

The chapter starts with a brief history of the virus, explaining when it was first identified and what commonly-used words connected with the virus actually mean. The chapter then goes on to explain what effects HIV can have on the body, when the effects become diagnosed as AIDS and how tests can identify that the immune system has been impaired.

The next section explains how HIV can and cannot be transmitted, some basic information on risk reduction[2] and how basic health and safety procedures, 'universal precautions', are amply sufficient to avoid HIV infection in most occupational settings.

Towards the end of the chapter statistics are given to provide a broad overview of the demographic features of people with HIV and AIDS. The chapter ends with cautious optimism about the medical developments in the treatment and containment of the HIV virus but stresses, however, that it is still equally important to address the discrimination faced by people who are affected.

About HIV and AIDS: A Brief History

In 1981 doctors in the USA began reporting cases of highly unusual infections and diseases among otherwise healthy young men. Two particular features of those reported cases gave a small group of doctors cause for concern. First, they were seeing types of infections or diseases rarely seen before among that age group or population. Second, the *severity* of those diseases or infections was astonishing. In fact, in the beginning, patients were sometimes dying before the doctors had a chance to engage in comprehensive study or diagnosis.

Compounding the confusion was the fact that nearly all of the early cases were among gay men or intravenous drug users. Researchers struggled to determine the cause of this new cluster of diseases and understand more fully its effects.

When reported cases began to include haemophiliacs (who must use blood products to stay healthy) and people who were the recipients of blood transfusions, the connection became increasingly obvious. It seemed that blood and other bodily fluids with a white blood cell count were responsible for transmission of this new disease. It also became clear that somehow the immune system of patients had been dangerously compromised; people were becoming ill and dying from *secondary* infections that resulted from a *primary* collapse of the body's natural defences.

It appeared that all of the people who were becoming ill with this disease were infected with a virus that acted directly on the body's immune system, rendering it sometimes helpless against common and uncommon diseases and infections. That virus was eventually isolated and (after considerable debate) named the Human Immunodeficiency Virus (HIV). Around the same time a name for the conditions associated with HIV came into consistent usage. It was AIDS, Acquired Immune Deficiency Syndrome.

The name itself reveals a lot about the condition. It is 'Acquired' because people 'get it' by engaging in specific behaviours with HIV infected persons; it does not 'just happen' and it is not spread through casual contact. It is 'Immune deficiency' because it depletes the strength of the body's immunity. And it is a 'Syndrome' because it is not just one sign or symptom; instead, it manifests itself as a number of secondary symptoms, diseases and infections that result from immunosuppression.

Finally, researchers began to note that some people with AIDS had probably been carrying HIV for a long time (sometimes years) before they became ill, while others became ill comparatively soon (six months or less) after infection with HIV had presumably occurred. During the time that patients had been *infected* but free of overt symptoms, they had also been *infectious*; capable of passing HIV to others through specific behaviours. This realisation was disturbing and frightening, since it meant that people could look and feel healthy and still transmit the virus. It also raised the question, which has not yet been fully answered, of how many of those who were infected, but asymptomatic, would go on to develop AIDS or AIDS related illness over the course of time.

What Does HIV Do?

Largely because of media reporting, the general public is accustomed to thinking strictly in terms of 'AIDS' itself as the sole cause for concern. But 'AIDS' is only one dimension to being infected with HIV. Put simply, what actually happens is as follows.

People acquire the virus through very specific sexual and blood-sharing activities. At this point the person is termed 'HIV antibody positive', 'HIV+', 'HIV seropositive' or 'HIV-infected'. All of the terms mean the same thing.

When a person acquires the virus, the body does not show external signs of being infected straight away. Instead,

HIV 'hides', waiting sometimes many years to take direct action against the immune system. The fact that the body has been generating an antibody that attempts to ward off HIV is insufficient by itself because that antibody is ultimately ineffective against HIV.

The term 'co-factors' indicates something else has to take place before the virus is effectively 'activated'. Co-factors are not the same as the behaviours that led to infection in the first place. For example, poor nutrition or high levels of chemical use may be common co-factors that explain why one person harbouring a virus becomes ill, while another does not. HIV *may* act in the same way. Typical advice to people newly diagnosed as HIV positive is to reduce stress, decrease or eliminate chemical or alcohol use, have plenty of rest and improve diet and exercise regimes. All or some of these things may be significant co-factors explaining why some people who are HIV positive become ill and others seem to remain perfectly healthy for a very long time. Research, however, is still not conclusive about what may 'trigger' viral activity in the case of HIV.

If HIV has become activated and immunity is depleted, then people may become ill with a number of 'opportunistic' infections ('opportunistic' indicates that they are infections that 'seize the opportunity' of weakened immunity in order to take hold). Common opportunistic infections associated with HIV related illness include: Pneumocystis Carinii pneumonia (or PCP), a rare form of parasitic pneumonia that leaves the patient with a persistent fever, dry cough and shortness of breath; and Kaposi's sarcoma (or KS), a rare form of cancer that is usually signalled by a purplish rash with lesions. Other infections include:

- Candidiasis (commonly known as thrush), a fungal infection in the mouth or oesophagus;

- Cryptosporidiosis, an infection caused by a parasite that lodges in the intestines, causing severe diarrhoea;

- Cytomegalovirus (CMV), a virus that causes mild to severe flu-like symptoms;

- Herpes zoster (commonly known as shingles) which are small and painful blisters on the skin that follow nerve pathways;
- Lymphadenopathy, an enlargement of the lymph nodes in the neck or groin; and
- Toxoplasmosis, a parasite infection that generates fevers and other symptoms.

When Does HIV Become AIDS?

When people develop one or more of the symptoms described above, or other symptoms related to HIV, does this mean they have moved from an HIV positive diagnosis to having AIDS?

The answer is, not necessarily. In order to have an epidemiological diagnosis of AIDS itself, the individual must evidence a number of particular infections or cancers. The diagnostic guidelines have, in fact, changed several times since the beginning of the epidemic and are likely to change again in the future. Women with HIV, for example, have experienced a number of gynaecological complications related to immunosuppression that for many years were not included within official diagnostic criteria for AIDS. The definitions are therefore imperfect.

Between the point when people are first infected with HIV and the point when they meet the case definition for a diagnosis of AIDS, there is a wide range of clinical possibilities. Since there are myriad opportunistic infections – some relatively 'mild' and other comparatively severe – and since individuals with HIV infections could be experiencing any possible combination of those infections, it would be most accurate to refer to a 'spectrum of infection' when talking about how people with HIV do and do not become ill.

In other words, if asymptomatic HIV seropositivity were placed at one end of a continuum and 'has AIDS and is currently extremely ill' were placed at the other end, people with HIV infection could fall anywhere along the continuum. The 'spectrum of infection' reveals that AIDS is not an 'either/or disease', but a range of conditions related to HIV infection. It is impossible to predict to what degree, *if at all*, people with asymptomatic HIV infection will 'progress' along the spectrum of infections, or what specific opportunistic infections, if any, they will experience.

Even when a person has been given a medical diagnosis of AIDS, it does not necessarily tell us about the individual's present condition or well-being. People have been diagnosed with cancer, for example, and have then experienced long periods of remission during which they felt and functioned normally.

HIV and AIDS can work the same way. A person may be diagnosed with AIDS because of a bout of PCP, for example, and upon recovery feel fine, look fine and remain healthy for months or even years afterwards, but the diagnosis of AIDS still remains.

A Note on Terminology

Because there is such a wide spectrum of conditions related to HIV, in most parts of this book reference is made to 'people with HIV related illnesses' or 'conditions'. Using such terms avoids having to make imperfect distinctions between having or not having AIDS.

How Can Immune Impairment be Identified?

The extent to which the immune system has been damaged by HIV can be measured by certain medical tests.

The 'CD4 count' is, as its name implies, a measurement of CD4 cells (also known as T4 cell count). CD4 cells are a type of white blood cell important to the body's immune system. HIV infection results in a loss of CD4 cells, reducing the immune system's ability to fight off infection.

An occasional low CD4 count does not necessarily mean the immune system is damaged: it may just, for example, mean you are recovering from a recent illness. The CD4 test can only give significant results if it is administered over a period of time. A *persistently* low CD4 count (below 500) indicates that the immune system is weakened. If the count falls below 200 there is increased likelihood of serious infections. It is usually below the 200 point that people with HIV are advised to consider taking drugs to combat the effects of HIV.

The CD4 test has been criticised for not really being able to predict good health: some people with low CD4 counts seem to remain perfectly healthy for long periods of time.

More recently developed tests which aim to determine when, and what type of, treatments should be given to people who are HIV positive are the 'viral load tests'. These tests can measure the number of virus particles per cubic millimetre of blood.

The viral load tests have been criticised because different versions of the tests seem to give different results about the same blood. They have also been criticised because they can only measure the level of the virus in the *blood*, which contains only a small proportion of the total viral load in the body.

Because, at the time of writing, viral load tests are relatively new there may be modifications and improvements to the tests in the future.

How HIV is Transmitted

Despite public confusion, there is solid reliable information about how HIV is transmitted and how it is not. Mass media reporting on transmission has not always put the facts about transmission into proper perspective. In some instances it has detailed extremely rare cases as if they were commonplace. Understanding a few basic principles of transmission helps to balance the picture.

1. HIV is a very fragile virus. Once outside the human body, it does not live very long at all, generally no more than several minutes. Whilst inside the body the virus can be very powerful, once it is exposed to the environment it is essentially deactivated in a very short period of time. This is not to indicate that if you should encounter spilled blood, you should estimate the amount of time it has been there before

touching it. Universal precautions should always be observed (see later).

2. HIV has to effectively 'get out of' one body and 'get into' another body before the necessary preconditions for transmission are met. Fortunately this is somewhat difficult to accomplish for two reasons. First, intact skin is a perfect barrier and, even if HIV infected blood were to come into direct contact with unbroken skin, it would be extremely difficult for the virus to pass through into the body and cause infection. Second, HIV is not an airborne virus. It is not passed by coughing, sneezing or breathing the same air as an HIV infected person.

3. Despite the fact that common advice has warned people against sharing 'bodily fluids', the reality is that there are only a few specific bodily fluids that have been implicated in HIV transmission. They are blood, semen, vaginal secretions (meaning the lubrication inside a woman's vagina, and not menstrual blood, which would be included under 'blood'), and to a much lesser degree, breast milk. The virus has been detected in bodily fluids such as saliva, but the amount of HIV therein is simply not sufficient for transmission.

HIV is not easy to acquire. Transmission requires certain specific behaviours or actions. In short, HIV is not spread by casual contact of any kind: touching, shaking hands, kissing (since kissing by itself is extremely unlikely to involve an exchange of blood, semen or vaginal secretions), and other contact. Nor is it spread by coughing or sneezing, sharing combs, eating utensils, towels or soap. Uninfected people can safely use the same showers, baths, and toilets as infected people. In addition there has never been any danger from mosquitoes or other insects or animals.

What is not safe, and what has been implicated in nearly every single case of HIV infection, is a small set of blood-sharing and unprotected sexual activities. They include:

1. Vaginal intercourse.

2. Anal intercourse.

3. Oral sex in some situations: the act of swallowing infected semen, blood or vaginal secretions is not what transmits HIV, enzymes in the stomach kill the virus; one would have to have an opening of some kind in the mouth in order for HIV to enter the body and potentially infect.

4. Pregnancy, from an HIV antibody positive mother to baby. There have been several documented cases of HIV transmission linked to breast milk, but there have also been a number of cases of HIV infected mothers breast-feeding their babies without infection taking place. This is an area which requires more study. In the meantime HIV positive mothers are advised not to breast-feed.

5. Needle-sharing and the sharing of other drug injection equipment. (It is certainly possible, of course, that sharing needles for other purposes could transmit HIV. Blood-sharing rituals, such as brother/sister pacts, or the use of unsterilised needles for tattooing or body piercing could potentially result in infection. No cases have been reported to date, however.)

The degree to which the preceding activities and behaviours have been implicated in HIV transmission allows us to assert that if we could alter the sexual and injecting behaviour of everyone in the UK, the transmission of HIV would virtually stop.

HIV Transmission: Risk Reduction

To prevent HIV infection, individuals must choose from among a range of specific strategies, each of which presents some difficulty. Since there is no danger of HIV infection from casual contact, we will address those behaviours – sex and drug use – known to be risk factors for HIV acquisition.

1. Individuals can choose not to have oral, vaginal, or anal sex. As a strategy this is often recommended, but it has its shortcomings. If one has already had unprotected intercourse, for example, she or he may already be HIV infected. And many tend to hear the recommendation of abstinence as a short-term commitment; in the context of HIV prevention, abstinence as a strategy means that one will not have oral, vaginal, or anal sex with anyone until a successful vaccine is made available, which may be many years away. For many people such a commitment is understandably impossible to make. It is critical, especially when talking to adolescents, who tend to view time in spans of weeks and months rather than years and decades, to be clear about the meaning of abstinence as a risk-reduction strategy for HIV infection.

2. Individuals can enter into a monogamous relationship and avoid sex with anyone other than their primary partner. For many people, this strategy will work quite well. But again, it needs to be clarified. Monogamy as a risk-reduction strategy for the prevention of HIV infection implies two things:

   (a) Neither partner has had unprotected sex or shared drug injection equipment with anyone before. The oft-heard statement contending that 'every time you have sex with someone you're also having sex with everyone they've had sex with, and so on' is absolutely true.

   (b) The relationship will last, and remain monogamous until a successful vaccine is developed. As an ideal, this is certainly sincere; no one enters into a committed relationship thinking it will only last a short duration. Despite best intentions, however, relationships do end, and marriages end in divorce. Many people in our society tend to practise what is termed 'serial monogamy', that is, they are faithful to their current partners even though they may have a number of partners over their lifetime. Serial monogamy is not the same as strict monogamy when it comes to HIV prevention.

3. If individuals choose to be sexually active, they can reduce their risk of HIV infection by practising safer sex. Safer sex indicates two things:

   (a) Sexual activity, such as fondling or mutual masturbation, that does not involve the exchange of blood, semen or vaginal secretions; or

   (b) The correct use of a latex condom or other effective barrier every time one has intercourse.

   Condoms are not foolproof. They do not eliminate risk, but they can help to reduce it significantly. The key to their effectiveness is proper use, and use every time one has intercourse. For some people, such consistency is difficult. For many, condoms seem awkward, embarrassing or uncomfortable. Even the thought of having to buy them in a chemist, where one knows the assistant, can be enough to deter their use. But for those people, and there are many, unable or unwilling to adhere to abstinence or strict monogamy, safer sex is the most effective tool available against HIV infection.

4. Individuals can avoid injecting drugs, or, at the very least, avoid sharing drug injection equipment. It may appear on the surface hypocritical even to mention a strategy that sounds like 'safe injectable drug use', and can put the drug/alcohol abuse educator in an uncomfortable position. Nevertheless, there are people injecting heroin, cocaine, methadone and other drugs who cannot or will not, for the moment, discontinue use. For them our best hope is to keep them free of life-threatening conditions such as AIDS so that they might live to someday seek help or treatment.

5. Individuals can avoid mixing any drug or alcohol use with sexual activity. Even armed with a good 'plan' for HIV risk reduction, it has been noted that chemical use impairs judgement and diminishes one's capacity to adhere to prearranged commitments.

There are a few strategies, some commonly presented, that simply do not work to prevent HIV infection:

1. Having sex only with 'people I know' or 'people from good backgrounds'. The truth is that anyone who has engaged in certain behaviours with an HIV infected person can, themselves, become HIV infected. Behaviourally, HIV is a democratic virus.

2. Asking people to disclose their sexual or drug-taking history. As a strategy this only encourages people to withhold the truth and is, at the least, extremely uncomfortable or embarrassing for most. In addition, it leads to the presumption that someone who has had multiple sexual partners is infected, and someone who has not is not. Only the HIV antibody test can determine with any accuracy an individual's HIV status.

3. Having the HIV antibody test. There are many reasons why one might rationally consider being tested, but it is important to note that having the test, by itself, does nothing to prevent HIV infection. The test is a diagnostic instrument, not a risk-prevention strategy.

Making choices among the available options is a very personal responsibility. For some, abstinence will prove to be the only viable alternative. Others may choose to have intercourse, but use condoms. The only way individuals can make a reasonable decision is by weighing all the available facts and measuring them against their own values, beliefs and traditions.

Universal Precautions

For most organisations, whether in the private, statutory or independent sector, there is little risk of occupational HIV infection – even in settings where individuals come into contact with blood or other infectious bodily fluids. Even so, some precautions are desirable. In fact, good infection control is wise even in the absence of HIV: it can help to reduce common diseases and infections (colds, flu, and so forth) that tend to spread rapidly through workplaces.

It is essential that each organisation investigates and checks that its procedures relating to health and safety, including standard good procedures for infection control, are up to date and relevant to the current workforce and are in operation. However, a few basics of infection control can be summarised as follows.

1. Always assume that everybody is potentially infectious for HIV and hepatitis. Because of the limits of technology in relation to testing, no one can ever be certain who is infected and who is not. Infection practices should, therefore, be implemented in every single case. This approach is called 'universal precautions'.

2. All employees should avoid direct contact with blood, semen and vaginal secretions (and in the case of hepatitis, saliva as well). Practically, most employees will only encounter risk in the case of accidental injuries – cuts, for example, that produce bleeding.

3. If contact with potentially infectious bodily fluids is necessary, latex gloves will provide an impermeable barrier. It should be noted that even infected blood on unbroken skin cannot cause infection; HIV has to get inside the body.

4. Common household bleach kills HIV and will be an efficient disinfectant.

5. Good general hygiene and workplace cleanliness are sensible in any case. Regular hand washing will help to reduce the number of common infections (colds, flu, etc.) that tend to spread through the workplace. It should also be kept in mind that because of suppressed immunity, people without HIV infection pose a greater threat to people with HIV infection than vice versa. In the interests of continued good health for people with HIV, the organisation should be kept clean and free of all possible exposure to bacteria, fungi and viruses.

In the end, a level-headed approach to infection control is best. There is no reason to over-react because HIV is difficult to transmit. Occupational transmission is extremely rare even among healthcare workers. But the presence of HIV and hepatitis provide organisations with an opportunity to re-evaluate their approach to healthy workplaces in general.

How Widespread is HIV? A Few Statistics

Any book which gives figures about how many people have HIV and AIDS will, of course, become out of date as soon as new figures are produced. The aim in this section is only to give an idea of the number of people with HIV and AIDS and, more significantly, to give some idea of the groups of people who are most affected and to identify any trends connected to this.[3]

HIV is indeed a serious, world-wide problem. By June 1996 world-wide figures for the reported number of people diagnosed as having AIDS had risen to 1,393,649. This figure seriously underestimates the true total number of cases because of the number of cases which are undiagnosed or unreported. The number in the world who are infected with HIV may be many times this number. The figure is impossible to estimate, however, because world-wide many people are not tested for HIV at least until the condition of AIDS is suspected – if, that is, they are ever tested at all.

In the UK, since reporting began in 1982, to the end of 1996, there were 28,447 people known to have been infected with HIV. In the same period, 13,720 people were reported to have been diagnosed as having developed AIDS and, of these, 9678 (71%) are known or presumed to have died.[4]

How Did People Become Infected?

World-wide the main way that HIV and AIDS have been transmitted is by heterosexual sex. In affluent western countries the majority of people with HIV and AIDS, to date, have been men who acquired the virus through having sex with other men. Trends clearly show, however, that the proportion of men newly infected by male sexual intercourse is decreasing while the number of people infected by other means is increasing. In 1986, for example, 94% of the cases of AIDS reported that year were attributable to sex between men, 1% to sex between men and women and 2% to injecting drug use. In mid 1996, 69% of the cases of AIDS reported were attributable to sex between men, 23% to sex between men and women and 7% to injecting drug use.[5]

Who Has HIV Affected? – Sex, Sexuality, Ethnicity and Age

A growing number of women[6] and heterosexual men are becoming infected with HIV. In mid 1996 over 15% of the total number of people infected with HIV were women and 67% of these women were infected by heterosexual sex. Figures for men showed 21% were infected by other means than male to male sex and, of these, 40% were infected by heterosexual sex.[7]

Although it is very important to recognise that year by year a growing proportion of people are contracting HIV by heterosexual sex or injecting drugs; it is equally important not to lose sight of the fact that the cumulative figures (the total number of cases since recording began) still show that sex between men accounts for 73% of all cases of AIDS and 61% of all known cases of HIV infection.[8]

The above point is crucial for underlining the fact that, of all the communities affected, gay and bisexual men have borne the brunt of the epidemic in the UK.

Although figures are not available for the percentage of people infected by HIV who are from black or ethnic minorities, some figures are available about the ethnicity of people with AIDS. By June 1996, nearly 17% of people with a diagnosis of AIDS whose ethnicity was known defined themselves as Black, Asian, Oriental, mixed race or from a category other than white;[9] of these, 34% were women and 28% were gay or bisexual men.

The age range of people affected by HIV and AIDS is generally much lower than most other long-term illnesses or conditions such as cancer or heart disease. In fact, 89% of people with HIV and, of those, 80% who have AIDS, are under 45 years of age and 21% of people with HIV are under 25 years of age.

Looking Forward to the Future

At the time of writing there is still no cure for HIV infection. There is no drug or combination of drugs which can erase HIV from the body or repair the damage that HIV has done to the immune system.

Since the advent of HIV, however, there have been considerable advances in the treatment and prevention of the illnesses and conditions that people develop as a result of HIV. *More and more people with HIV are responding to treatments, remaining well for longer periods and living longer lives.*

In addition, there is considerable optimism in the medical profession and amongst those working with HIV, that we are closer and closer to the point where HIV can be kept under control by a combination of different drugs and treatments.

Treatments are expensive and, as a world-wide problem, there are many hurdles to be overcome before we could even imagine that HIV could cease to be a threat to humankind. Compared with the seemingly hopeless situation of the early 1980s, however, there is at least cause to celebrate the progress that has been made to date.

The Need to Take Action in the Workplace

Even though many people with HIV can expect to remain well for longer and live longer lives, there is one problem that people with HIV face that has not gone away – discrimination. The workplace has been a major area where people have suffered discrimination and this is an important reason why workplace initiatives are needed in relation to HIV and AIDS.

Faced with the facts about HIV and AIDS – particularly

the modes of transmission – there is clearly no scientific basis for segregation, isolation, discrimination or second-rate provision for people affected. Unfortunately, the rationale for discrimination is fear, not fact.

For people with HIV, the combined effects of trying to come to terms with a possibly fatal condition and at the same time suffering the effects of discrimination can be practically, emotionally and psychologically devastating.

2 HIV and Employment Law

This chapter looks at employment law in the UK in relation to HIV. For people who are HIV positive and have no symptoms related to their HIV status, there is no specific employment law which gives protection against discrimination. There are, however, a number of statutory employment rights which give a degree of protection to all employees. The government has also issued guidelines to employers which state that people affected by HIV should not be treated differently from other employees.

People who are HIV positive and have or have had symptoms or illnesses related to their condition are now protected, in some circumstances, by the employment provisions of the Disability Discrimination Act which took effect in December 1996.

The chapter begins by describing the statutory employment laws which give rights to all employees regardless of their HIV status. It goes on to show how these laws relate to people who are HIV positive. Chapter 3 explains how people who are HIV positive and symptomatic may be covered by the Disability Discrimination Act.

Statutory Employment Law and HIV

Terms and Conditions

With few exceptions, all employees who work eight or more hours a week for more than a month are entitled to a statutory statement of their main terms and conditions of employment within two months of starting work. The statement should include:

- the name of employer and employee;
- date of starting work;
- job title or a brief description of the job;
- place(s) of work;
- details of pay (the amount due and when) and hours of work.

Plus any terms and conditions relating to: incapacity for work due to sickness or injury; holiday entitlement and holiday pay; pensions (in some circumstances only); length of notice required by both employer and employee.

If there are no particulars to give (for example, because there is no pension or sick pay scheme) then the statement must say so.

Disciplinary and Grievance Procedures

The written statement must also specify any disciplinary rules which apply to the employee and give details of the disciplinary and grievance procedures. It must also mention (by description or name) (i) the person to whom an employee can apply if they are dissatisfied with the decision of a disciplinary procedure and (ii) a person to contact to resolve a grievance. If the disciplinary and grievance procedures are not detailed in the written statement, the statement should refer to a document which does contain them.

Any changes to these terms have to be notified individually to each employee.

Dismissals

The Employment Protection (Consolidation) Act 1978 requires that employers must have a prescribed reason and be reasonable in sacking under the meaning of the Act. This means that employees who believe their employer has acted unreasonably in sacking them can take a case of 'unfair dismissal' to an industrial tribunal. However, there is a qualifying period needed to take a case, i.e. to claim 'unfair dismissal' an employee must have been in continuous employment for two years or more with the same employer. (At the time of writing, the qualifying period is under review.)

Cases brought on the basis of sex, race or disability discrimination, trade union membership or for trying to assert a basic statutory right have no qualifying period. An employee claiming unfair dismissal must make a claim within three months of the dismissal. Employees claiming discrimination must claim within three months of the last act of discrimination taking place.

If the tribunal finds the dismissal unfair, the employer can be ordered to reinstate the employee or award compensation.

Constructive Dismissal

An employee who feels their employer has made their employment situation so difficult that they have to resign can also claim 'constructive dismissal', with the same qualifying periods. The employee should inform the employer in writing of the reasons why they are resigning if they intend to claim 'constructive dismissal' at a later stage. The law around 'constructive dismissal' is, however, extremely complicated.

Wrongful Dismissal

A qualifying period of employment is not required to claim 'wrongful dismissal'. In deciding whether or not an employee has been wrongfully dismissed a court or industrial tribunal must only consider if there has been a breach of contract by the employer. Whether an employer has acted reasonably is not relevant in cases of wrongful dismissal. If an employee wins a case of wrongful dismissal they are only entitled in most cases to their notice pay. Employers cannot be required to re-employ the worker.

How Do These Laws Relate to People Who are HIV and Asymptomatic?

In 1989 the Department of Employment and the Health and Safety Executive produced 'AIDS and the Workplace: A Guide for Employers'. The guidelines state:

> Dismissal purely on the basis that an employee is infected with HIV could be held to be unfair under the legislation.[1]

An employee who is HIV positive and asymptomatic would usually have to have the two year qualifying period in order to claim unfair dismissal at an industrial tribunal. There is, however, a possibility of male employees taking a case of HIV discrimination on the grounds of indirect sex discrimination because there are more men who are HIV positive than women. If a case were to be taken on the grounds of sex discrimination, no qualifying period of employment would be needed. To date, such a case has not been tested in law.

In certain circumstances the Race Relations Act could be used in relation to HIV. It is unlawful for an employer to lay down conditions which do not apply to employees of different racial groups. For example, it is illegal for an employer to only ask people of a certain race, nationality or ethnic origin to take an HIV test.

Harassment and Victimisation

Within every contract of employment there is an implied duty of trust and confidence for both employer and employee. Past tribunal cases have established that harassment or victimisation of an employee by the employer or other employees can be considered as a breach of mutual trust and confidence.

An employer's duty of care towards an employee who is HIV positive or thought to be will entail taking steps to prevent or avoid harassment by co-workers. Failure to provide support might justify the employee resigning and claiming constructive dismissal.

Another important point is that the Criminal Justice and Public Order Act 1994 has introduced a new offence of intentional harassment on the grounds of race, sex, sexuality, age and disability. The Act includes harassment in the workplace. Employees who are harassed by work colleagues or by their employer are now in a position to report the matter to the police.

Pressure to Dismiss

Government advice and tribunal cases also suggest that employers who dismiss someone affected by HIV because of pressure to do so by other employees, would not be regarded as reasonable under employment law: pressure to dismiss an employee backed by a strike or threat of a strike should be ignored as stated in the Employment Protection (Consolidation) Act 1978, Section 63.

The very least an employer is expected to do in these circumstances is to investigate the complaints to discover the cause of the problem and to consider ways of dealing with it. Employees who do harass or refuse to work with people affected by HIV may well be in breach of contract themselves and could therefore face disciplinary action and even criminal charges.

Tribunal Cases

There are very few cases involving HIV or AIDS which have reached an industrial tribunal. In those that have, the responsibility of the employers to follow proper investigation and procedures has been stressed. All of the following cases took place in the 1980s and all involve assumptions by colleagues that an employee was HIV positive simply because of the fact that he was gay.

In *Buck* v. *Letchworth Palace Ltd* (1987) Mr Buck was sacked because his fellow employees refused to work with him. Mr Buck had been employed as a projectionist for 17 years when in November 1986 he was convicted for a second time of importuning in a public lavatory. Management already knew Mr Buck was gay and about his previous conviction but had previously taken no action. On this occasion, however, two part-time projectionists and the cinema manager decided that Mr Buck's way of life exposed him to the risk of 'catching AIDS' and they feared that they might catch it from him. Because of this, he was sacked.

The industrial tribunal upheld the decision as fair. The case went to the Employment Appeals Tribunal (EAT) who advised that the employer should pay compensation. The EAT decision was based on the fact that the company had not held a proper inquiry.

In *Cormack* v. *TNT Sealion Ltd* (1986) crew members refused to work with a chef on board ship. The complaint to personnel was initially understood to be one relating to the personal hygiene of Mr Cormack. It transpired, however, that the real reason was because he was gay and suspected of having AIDS. The management transferred Mr Cormack to another ship. Unfortunately a situation arose in the new ship where he and other crew members were made redundant. The tribunal found that the dismissal was fair on the grounds that the employer had scrupulously followed its selection criteria for redundancy. However, the tribunal commented:

> The innuendo behind the complaints of lack of personal hygiene is that Mr Cormack was a homosexual and suspected carrier of the AIDS virus and this led to an unjustified and emotional reaction against him by the Chief Officer. This is a problem that is likely to arise with increasing frequency and a good employer who is fair to his employees must be seen to act promptly to lay to rest all unfounded suspicions. He has an obligation to safeguard the health and safety of his employees on the one hand which must be balanced against his obligations to deal fairly with the individual employee on the other.

The tribunal suggested that if the dismissal had been on the basis of unfounded complaints about a homosexual employee and AIDS, without any proper investigation or inquiry, then they would have approached the case in a completely different way. The tribunal suggested that in such a situation the employer should investigate the complaints and inform the employee immediately.

In *Philpott and Adelaja* v. *North Lambeth Law Centre* (1987) two solicitors at North Lambeth Law Centre objected to the recruitment of another solicitor because he was gay and they thought he would therefore have AIDS. After an internal inquiry both were sacked and an industrial tribunal found their dismissal fair.

Although there are few related tribunal cases, many people affected by HIV have had problems in employment. One of the reasons why there have been so few cases is that many were settled out of court, or an employer offered a sum of money on termination of employment which was more than the tribunal was likely to award as compensation. In many other cases related to HIV, however, employees have not pursued cases because of the fear that publicity surrounding a case may expose them to further discrimination in other areas of life.

Providing Information

Laws relating to health and safety are another area which the employer should be aware of. Under Section 2 of the Health and Safety at Work Act, employers have a duty to provide adequate information, instruction and training to their workforce. This is also part of their common law duty of care. Under these laws, employers may well have a duty to provide information about HIV and its modes of transmission. 'AIDS and the Workplace: A Guide for Employers' states:

> All companies, large or small, should provide information on AIDS and the workplace. Larger companies should consider implementing an education programme.[2]

HIV Testing and Employment: Recruitment

There is no law to stop employers asking for an HIV antibody test as part of a company medical for all new recruits. But employers and/or company doctors must obtain the new recruit's express consent to be tested for HIV antibodies. Doctors who conduct the test without a person's consent risk criminal charges of assault if they take the blood specimen and civil liability for assault and battery.

The employer does not have the right to know the test results, but can refuse an offer of employment if the individual refuses to give permission for the test or disclosure of the results. In order for the employer to know the results of the test, the individual must give consent for the doctor to disclose the results to the employer.

In the UK we have a somewhat bizarre situation that an employer can refuse employment if a test has been taken and showed positive, but only if there are no symptoms or illnesses related to the individual's status which are known to the employer. Chapter 3 explains why it would usually be illegal, under the Disability Discrimination Act, to discriminate against someone who had, or had had, an HIV related illness but was capable of undertaking the job applied for.

As with dismissal, there is a potential case for any male job applicants to claim indirect sex discrimination if they are refused employment because they are HIV positive. To date, this has not been tested in law.

It is worth noting that in 1987 the Equal Opportunities Commission (EOC) investigated Dan Air for only employing female cabin staff. Part of Dan Air's reason for this was that they maintained that a large number of men attracted to be cabin staff were homosexual and therefore more likely to have AIDS.

The EOC rejected Dan Air's arguments and concluded their investigation by issuing a non-discriminatory notice. The notice required Dan Air to open employment to men and to make changes in their recruitment, interviewing and selection process. Training in sex discrimination was also recommended. Although the Dan Air investigation did not involve HIV testing, the results of the investigation could be cited if a case was brought against an employer who tested at recruitment.

Testing Existing Employees

The only way that an employer can insist on existing employees being tested for HIV antibodies is if the initial terms and conditions of service stated that this would be the case for the employee. Otherwise the employer is liable to claims of constructive dismissal, a claim for damages, breach of contract or wrongful dismissal.

Considerations which should be taken into account in regard to workplace HIV antibody testing are explored in detail in Chapter 5.

Confidentiality

In relation to employment law, it is the previously mentioned implicit contractual duty of mutual trust and confidence which gives some protection concerning confidentiality. The duty of trust and confidence includes a duty for both employer and employee not to disclose confidential information obtained in the course of employment.

Employers are not legally entitled to disclose that an employee is infected with HIV unless the employee consents. The only exception to this rule is if it could be claimed that it was in the public interest for others to know – this is a standard defence to breach of confidence claims.

Confidentiality and workplace issues are discussed in more detail in Chapter 4.

Employment in Healthcare

Although employment law is not different for people working in healthcare, it is useful to note the guidance from the medical profession in relation to people working with

HIV. It is important because healthcare is one of the very few areas where there may be reasons to be tested in some, albeit rare, cases.

The General Medical Council (GMC) has ruled that doctors and, by implication other health workers, with HIV infection are ethically obliged to seek professional advice on whether or not they need to limit or modify their practice to protect their patients. GMC guidance 'HIV and AIDS: the ethical considerations' states:

> ... it is imperative, both in the public interest and on ethical grounds, that any doctor who thinks they may have been infected with HIV should seek appropriate diagnostic testing and counselling and, if found to be infected, have regular medical supervision.
>
> Doctors who are HIV positive should also seek specialist advice on the extent to which they should limit their practice in order to protect their patients. Such advice will usually be obtained from a consultant in occupational health, who may in turn seek guidance, on an anonymous basis, from the UK Advisory Panel of the Expert Advisory Group on AIDS. Doctors must act upon that advice which, in some circumstances, would include a requirement not to practise or to limit their practise in certain ways. No doctor should continue in clinical practice merely on the basis of their own assessment of the risks to patients ...
>
> It is unethical for doctors who know or believe themselves to be infected with HIV to put patients at risk by failing to seek appropriate counselling or by failing to act upon it when given. Such behaviour may result in proceedings by the GMC which could lead to the restriction or removal of a doctor's registration if this were necessary to protect patients or the doctor's own health.[3]

The guidelines do make it clear, however, that the risk of a doctor who is HIV positive endangering a patient is 'very small'. When the 1995 edition of the guidelines was published, there was only one known case in the whole world of a healthcare worker transmitting HIV to patients, in the course of dental treatment. Therefore, although healthcare professionals should seek the prescribed specialist advice, in the vast majority of cases, no limitation is needed and there is no reason or obligation to inform the employer.

This chapter has attempted to give an overview of the general employment laws in the UK and to show how these laws have related or could relate to HIV and the workplace issues. The following chapter goes on to give more specific detail about the provision of the Disability Discrimination Act and how the circumstances in which people with HIV will be afforded protection.

3 Disability Discrimination, HIV and Related Illnesses

The Disability Discrimination Act 1995

To understand how the Disability Discrimination Act (DDA) relates to people who are HIV positive and symptomatic, it is useful know a little about the Act generally. This section gives a brief outline of the DDA before going on to look at how and when people who are HIV positive are covered by the Act. The outline is not intended to be a comprehensive or exhaustive guide to the Act.

The DDA gives disabled people rights in the areas of employment, getting goods and services and buying or renting land or property. We are going to concentrate primarily on the employment provisions of the Act whilst looking first at who is covered by the Act generally.

The DDA is quite specific in how it defines disability. The Act states that:

> ... a person has a disability ... if he has a physical or mental impairment which has a substantial and long term adverse effect on his ability to carry out normal day-to-day activities.

The Act states that the physical or mental impairment must be of long-term effect and it states that:

> the effect of an impairment is a long term effect if (a) it has lasted at least 12 months; (b) the period for which it lasts is likely to be at least 12 months; or (c) it is likely to last for the rest of the life of the person affected.

The Act also states:

> where an impairment ceases to have a substantial adverse effect on a person's ability to carry out normal day-to-day activities, it is to be treated as continuing to have that effect if that effect is likely to recur.

People with 'progressive conditions' are regarded as disabled under the Act providing that, as a result of the condition, the person has an impairment which has or has had an effect on their ability to carry out 'normal day-to-day activities'. However, the effect on day-to-day activities does not have to be a substantial effect. It is within the category of progressive conditions that people who are HIV positive and symptomatic are explicitly covered by the Act. Conditions such as cancer, muscular dystrophy and multiple sclerosis are also covered in this category.

The Emphasis of UK Legislation

A major feature of the DDA is that it stresses medical models of disability rather than social models. The approach is such that people must usually experience 'a problem' with their disability before they are given legal protection. In contrast, a social approach to discrimination recognises that the individual would not necessarily have a problem if the negative attitudes of others towards them were eradicated.

The laws in the USA are a good example of how a social model gives wider protection against discrimination. The Americans with Disabilities Act 1990 (ADA), recognises that the social attitudes in relation to disability can be as important as the disability itself. Under the ADA, it is recognised that people may suffer discrimination because they are perceived to be disabled as well as actually being disabled. Because of this, people are legally protected from HIV related discrimination whether or not they are positive and whether or not they have been ill as a result of their HIV status.

Groups of individuals and organisations who are trying to strengthen or change the DDA in Britain are campaigning to change the emphasis of the Act to one which gives legal redress against all types of discrimination in relation to disability. Because of this, anyone involved in the forward planning and development of policy in relation to disability would be well advised to consider what the effects of a change or strengthening of the law would be.

Employment Provisions

The employment provisions of the Act came into force in December 1996. A useful summary of the employment provisions of the DDA is given in the free leaflet 'A brief guide to the Disability Discrimination Act' DL40, which is issued on behalf of the Minister for Disabled People.[1]

To give more explanation of how the Act is to be interpreted, the government has also laid down regulations and issued guidance on matters to be taken into account concerning the definition of disability. A code of practice on disability discrimination in employment has also been issued.

Despite government guidance, there are still many areas which are largely unexplained in the Act and which will be 'grey' areas until tested by the courts and tribunals. Ultimately it will be caselaw which determines some of the more ambiguous parts of the Act and this may take many years to establish.

What Employers Will Have to Do

It is against the law for an employer to treat a disabled person less favourably than someone else because of their disability, unless there is good reason. This applies to all employment matters (including recruitment, training, promotion and dismissal). Employers will, however, still be able to recruit or promote the best person for the job.

In order to help a person to do the job, employers will have to look at what changes they could make to the workplace or to the way the work is done, and make any changes which are reasonable. Employers will be able to take into account how much the changes would cost, and to what extent the changes really would make a material difference to a disabled person when considering what is reasonable. Employers are not expected to make any changes which would break health and safety laws. In addition to employers, it is against the law for trade associations, trade unions and professional bodies to treat a disabled person less favourably than someone else.

Employers who are Exempt

The employment part of the Act does not apply to employers who employ fewer than 20 people. However, they are encouraged to follow good practice guidelines.

The Act does not apply to operational staff employed in the armed forces, the police, the prison service, the fire service or to anyone employed on board ships, hovercraft or aeroplanes.

Complaints About Discrimination

Disabled people who feel that their employer has discriminated against them will be able to complain to an industrial tribunal. They can ask ACAS (the Advisory Conciliation and Arbitration Service), or in Northern Ireland the LRA (Labour Relations Agency), to help them. This may mean that the complaint can be settled without an industrial tribunal hearing.

There is no qualifying period of employment needed to take a case of discrimination to an industrial tribunal. Claims must usually be made within three months of the discrimination taking place.

The Act explicitly outlaws victimisation of disabled people. Any victimisation of or discrimination against a disabled person is the employer's responsibility – regardless of whether or not it occurred with the employer's knowledge or approval. Unlike the Sex Discrimination Act and the Race Relations Act, however, the concept of 'indirect discrimination' does not apply under the DDA.

We now go on to look at some key words in the Act, their legal meaning and their relevance to people who are HIV positive and symptomatic.

Protection in Relation to HIV

People who are HIV positive and symptomatic are treated as disabled under the Act provided that their illness or illnesses do have an effect (no matter how small) on their ability to carry out 'normal' day-to-day activities.

It is important to stress that people with progressive conditions which have yet to have any effect on their ability to carry out normal day-to-day activities are not covered by the Act.

The point at which a person who is HIV positive is defined as having symptoms or illnesses that have an effect on day-to-day activities may be a moot point. It will almost certainly be a matter for tribunals to decide based on the results of test cases and subsequent caselaw. For example, a person who is HIV positive may never have experienced any illness which is linked to their status. However, through regular hospital monitoring, they may find that they have a declining T-cell count indicating that they may be more vulnerable to certain infections. (T-Cells – T-lymphocytes – are white blood cells that play an important part in the immune system.) With a low T-cell count, it could be argued that there is an effect on day-to-day activities because there is a need to avoid overworking and stress-related situations in order to reduce the chances of infection. The question raised in this example is at what level would a tribunal accept that a count was low enough to have an effect on day-to-day activities?

Presumably medical opinion would be needed to establish if day-to-day work was affected in cases such as these.

Less Favourable Treatment

Recruitment. An employer will have a defence against a discrimination claim only if they can justify that the less favourable treatment of a disabled person was for a reason which is 'material to the circumstances of the particular case' and 'substantial'. That is, the employer must show that the reason for treating a disabled person differently was genuinely relevant in a given situation.

For example, an employer who rejects outright a job applicant because they disclose on their application form that they have had an HIV related illness would not usually have a defence for their actions. The employer would have a defence, however, if they could show that being HIV positive and symptomatic was genuinely relevant to the post applied for. Another defence may be that susceptibility to the particular HIV related illness experienced was also directly relevant to the job applied for.

It should be stressed, however, that the circumstances are extremely rare when an employer could argue that having had an HIV related illness was a genuine reason for not employing someone. In addition, it would not be sufficient to argue that the applicant had been rejected because they were highly likely to become ill or even seriously ill in the future.

Victimisation and Harassment. People who are HIV positive have experienced a unique form of discrimination because of the prejudice and misunderstanding about HIV.

Under the DDA, people who are HIV positive and symptomatic can now take claims of discrimination to an industrial tribunal if they are being discriminated against or have been sacked because of their status.

It is the employer's duty to ensure that discrimination does not occur. It is therefore in the employer's interest to ensure that other employees do not victimise, harass or discriminate in any way against colleagues who are HIV positive and symptomatic.

If an employee does experience discrimination because of their HIV status, the employer must take effective action against that discrimination to avoid claims against them.

Before the passing of the DDA, some people who were being discriminated against on the grounds of their HIV status were reluctant to take their case to an industrial tribunal because of the fear of publicity. This is understandable considering the problems some people have had when their HIV status has become widely known.

Taking cases of discrimination under the DDA may help to overcome the problems individuals face in relation to publicity. The individual complaining to a tribunal can now ask the tribunal to make a restricted reporting order. If restricted reporting is granted by the tribunal, then certain (and sometimes all) details of the case cannot be reported by the press except for the tribunal's decision at the end of the case. Tribunals can make a restricted order if evidence of 'a personal nature' is to be heard about the person complaining. Medical and other intimate evidence which might 'reasonably assumed to be likely to cause significant embarrassment' to the person complaining will be accepted to be of a 'personal nature'.

The Law in Relation to HIV Related Illnesses

The DDA states that nothing in the employment part of the Act is to be taken to require an employer to treat a disabled person more favourably than he treats or would treat others within the organisation. The only exceptions to this are the provisions made in Section 6, the employer's duty to make reasonable adjustments, discussed later. Thus, an employer would not usually be expected to give a disabled person and, in this context, a person with an HIV related illness, more favourable sick leave provisions in the contract than they would for other employees. Before the DDA was passed, government guidelines 'AIDS and the Workplace' stated that:

> HIV infection alone does not affect people's ability to do their job until they develop illnesses that make them unfit ... If they later become ill, they should be treated like anyone else with a life-threatening illness. Only if their illness affects their ability to do the job should their employer seek medical advice.[2]

This advice will not have changed substantially since the passing of the DDA, with the exception that employers must now be able to show that they have considered, and where reasonable acted upon, any changes they could make to the workplace, the way the work is done and/or the possibility of a move to different duties. The later section, 'Employer's Duty to Make a Reasonable Adjustment' outlines what these duties may be in relation to HIV related illnesses. The likelihood of there being suitable alternative employment will depend largely on the size of the firm involved.

Ill Health Retirement and Dismissals

If a person is genuinely not able to continue to work for an employer, the most beneficial option for the employee is for the employer to offer some package of early retirement on ill health grounds. The package the employer is able to offer will, of course, depend on the size and resources of the organisation.

If dismissal is the only option, then legally the dismissal must come under one of two headings: either on health grounds after proper medical enquiry, or for poor attendance.

If a person is dismissed because they are unable to do the job, the employer must have sufficient evidence upon which to base the decision. This involves, preferably, both a report from the employee's doctor and an examination by a doctor on behalf of the employer.

If the employer makes a decision to dismiss on the grounds of poor attendance due to a succession of minor illnesses, this is a reason related to conduct. Therefore, the employee should be given warnings, as appropriate, and an opportunity to improve. After that, if there is no improvement or explanation then the employer is eventually entitled to decide that 'enough is enough'.

Employer's Duty to Make a Reasonable Adjustment

Section 6 of the DDA states that an employer must take reasonable steps to prevent any physical feature of the premises, or any working arrangements that are made, from causing a substantial disadvantage to a disabled person. Under Section 5 (2) an applicant can complain if they feel that they did not get a job for which they applied because the employer had failed to make a Section 6 adjustment.

The duty to make adjustments arises when a disabled person is placed at a substantial disadvantage as either a job applicant or as an employee. The duty to make adjustments would only arise if the employer knew that a disabled person was applying for a job and that the disabled candidate was at a substantial disadvantage due to the employer's failure to make adjustments in comparison with other candidates.

In Section 6 (3), the Act gives examples of the steps an employer may have to take in order to comply with the duty to make adjustments. The list is reprinted here so that we can go on to look at the ways in which these changes could be implemented for someone who is HIV positive and has or has had related conditions or illnesses. The examples are:

(a) making adjustments to premises;

(b) allocating some of the disabled person's duties to another person;

(c) transferring him to fill an existing vacancy;

(d) altering his working hours;

(e) assigning him to a different place of work;

(f) allowing him to be absent during working hours for rehabilitation, assessment or treatment;

(g) giving him, or arranging for him to be given, training;

(h) acquiring or modifying equipment;

(i) modifying instructions or reference manuals;

(j) modifying procedures for testing or assessment;

(k) providing a reader or supervisor;

(l) providing supervision.

The list refers to 'him' or 'his', as quoted, but the Act applies equally to male and female employees.

Reasonable Adjustment and HIV

In 1992 LAGER (Lesbian and Gay Employment Rights) published the pamphlet 'HIV & AIDS: Continued Employment Guidelines for Employers'. The guidelines suggest action that employers can take to ensure that people affected by long-term or intermittent illness can remain in employment. Planning in advance is stressed as the key to dealing with any situation where an employee has a long-term or intermittent illness. The pamphlet goes on to suggest some practical ways in which the employer can adapt the working conditions and environment in order to help an employee remain in employment. At the time of writing there was no law to enforce the guidelines, although policy and good employment practice were recommended by the government. The passing of the DDA means that many of the suggestions in the pamphlet will now be mandatory for employers at least to consider if they are to avoid claims of discrimination by employees affected.

Some of the guidelines in the pamphlet are reprinted or revised below to give an idea of how the requirements of Section 6 could be fulfilled for someone with an HIV related illness or, indeed, any other intermittent or long-term illness. The extent to which the guidelines can be implemented will depend on the size and resources of the organisation.

It should be stressed that these are only suggestions and should not be taken as a definitive account of the way in which the law will be interpreted. The suggestions are also made to provide a 'model' or 'ideal' of good practice which, regardless of legal considerations, organisations are encouraged to work towards.

One of the most important ways of working out a satisfactory agreement between employee and employer is to discuss the situation with the employee at all stages. After all, it is the employee who will have the most information about how their illness or condition affects their ability to work and their day-to-day life. Even when work patterns have been mutually agreed between employer and employee, it is important to have regular meetings to ensure that circumstances have not changed.

A Change in Duties

> *Section 6 (3) (b) allocating some of the disabled person's duties to another person; (c) transferring him to fill an existing vacancy; (e) assigning him to a different place of work; (g) giving him, or arranging for him to be given, training*

Before considering a change in duties or a change of post, it is important to note that the greater the awareness of other staff about issues of long-term illness and HIV related issues, the greater the likelihood of their co-operation if duties need to be modified. This highlights the importance of giving training and information to staff in advance, thereby preparing for situations which might arise in the workplace.

Some employees affected by an HIV related illness may be able to continue their existing duties, others may not. Equally important to consider, however, is that there may be additional tasks that the employee can undertake – not listed in the job description – which can be substituted for those the employee can no longer do.

The employee affected by long-term illness/HIV related illness is the person most likely to know what they are capable of continuing to do. In some cases, however, it may also be useful to encourage the employee to ask the advice of their doctor as to how much, and what type of, continued work is appropriate. In many instances there will only be a few parts of the job which prove impossible for the employee to continue. Components of jobs which involve high stress situations and parts of jobs which require heavy lifting or carrying are some of the most frequent duties which need to be removed for people with HIV related conditions.

After identifying tasks that the employee feels unable to continue, it is then useful to assess first, the amount of time spent in an average week needed to perform these tasks and, second, how essential these tasks are to the organisation as a whole.

These assessments allow the employer to gauge the amount of work that needs to be devolved to other staff.

It is important to note that any attempt to force staff into taking on additional duties or changing duties against their will would be seen as a change in their terms and conditions of employment. Such changes may therefore constitute a breach of contract by the employer if not mutually agreed by every employee concerned. Industrial action can also be avoided by planning in advance with the relevant trade unions.

Staff may wish to discuss any changes with their trade union representative. This approach should be encouraged or suggested by the employer if a spirit of mutual co-operation is to be fostered.

Additional Duties

If an employee with a long-term illness/HIV related condition is able to continue the same hours of work but has had certain tasks removed, then they may be able to take on new duties. In some cases this may mean a straightforward swap of tasks with other employees. Additional training may be needed to help the transition from one set of duties to another.

Another way of working out additional duties is to evaluate the employee's whole job in the context of organisational development. That is, by taking into account the employee's overall work history, with particular regard to qualifications and experience gained in other organisations, there may be scope for previously untapped skills to be used to develop their job in a new or different direction. Obviously a change in direction would have to be considered in the context of the primary aims of the organisation and its future plans and targets.

The advantage of this latter approach is that it can change a situation from one of perceived compromise to one which gives positive motivation and new direction for both the employee concerned and the organisation as a whole.

A Change to Working Hours

Section 6 (3) (d) altering his working hours

Some employees who develop long-term illnesses or disabilities may be able to continue their existing work but with a change or reduction in hours. Forward planning within an organisation can work out how flexible the organisation is able to be if any such requests are made. Working out possibilities for job share schemes is one example of an arrangement which can be of benefit to both employee and employer.

For some employees, a cut in hours may not be appropriate as the employee may be able to work all of their existing hours but at different times from the organisation's 'usual' working day. For example, some people who develop a long-term illness or disability may find that they are able to continue their hours if they are spread out over a longer period of time.

Allowing employees to work from home for a certain period of time or for a portion of the week may be useful in some cases; because of inaccessible public transport, for example, people who have developed restricted mobility may find travel to work more tiring or more difficult than previously.

Some people with or recovering from illness may benefit from having rest periods or a short sleep, for example, after lunch breaks. If possible, it is very useful if employers can provide a room where employees can be assured of peace and quiet while the rest is being taken. Clearly this suggestion will not be possible in some organisations but should at least be considered if it is.

If a reduction in hours and a reduction in pay is the only solution available to both employee and employer, then clearly the relevant trade union should be consulted at all points of negotiation.

Returning to Work After Illness

Some employees may want to and be able to return to work after a serious illness, but may not be able to work at full capacity immediately.

Flexible procedures which allow the employee to build up their strength slowly can be vital for the employee's return to full health.

Allowing the employee to work with reduced hours, allocating more time for specific tasks or restricting duties for a temporary period are examples of the ways that employers can be flexible.

Work targets, mutually agreed with the employee, can be set in the context of the illness. In many cases the employee will have been advised by their doctor/hospital as to whether or not they are fit to maintain full working duties.

Keeping Jobs Open

Many employers may argue that they simply cannot afford to keep jobs open for employees who are on sick leave for long periods of time. It is worth remembering, however, that many employers used the same argument about women and maternity leave until legislation was introduced. Since that legislation, it is now common to see job advertisements for temporary workers needed to fill in for women on maternity leave.

If an employee needs to be away from work for longer than their sick leave entitlement, it may be possible for the employer and employee to negotiate a period of time for the job to kept open for them. In some cases the employee will be able to get medical advice about the amount of time they need to cover.

Time Away from Work

> *Section 6 (3) (f) allowing him to be absent during working hours for rehabilitation, assessment or treatment*

Many people with HIV have experienced problems at work because they need time off to attend regular hospital appointments for check-ups or monitoring their health. Although the appointments may be once weekly or less, employers have become suspicious as to the amount of time being taken off and either suspect serious illness or malingering. Because of this, some employees have felt obliged to inform their employer of their HIV status and have then experienced discrimination as a result. Other employees not wanting to tell their employer about their HIV status have felt obliged to make up excuses as to why the time is needed.

It is to be hoped that the provisions of the DDA will go some way to help with this situation if employees know they have the right to time off for such appointments and so forth. However, it will not overcome the problem that many individuals will not want to inform their employer of their status. Nor will it be of any assistance to people who have not become ill as a result of their status but still need to attend regular appointments. In these instances it is company policy and practices which can help the employee to feel supported if such situations arise.

Time Off for Illness

If the employee does not feel confident to discuss the issues with their employer, they may feel pressured to continue working when they are ill and so risk making the illness worse.

Sometimes the employee may try to continue working because they feel they have too much to do to be able to take time off. The employer (and sometimes colleagues) needs to be sensitive to the health of the employee with the long-term illness – sometimes the employee may need to be gently persuaded to take some time off to avoid making themselves more ill. For example, using informed judgement, the employer may suggest the employee takes a 'long weekend'. Time away from work may be a sensitive matter for the employee concerned, particularly people who are very work-identified. In some cases the employee may benefit from counselling to assess the need for time off.

Modifications and Adaptations

Section 6 (3) (a) making adjustments to premises; (i) modifying instructions or reference manuals; (h) acquiring or modifying equipment; (j) modifying procedures for testing or assessment; (k) providing a reader or supervisor

Most people who have or have had HIV related illnesses do not develop physical disabilities as a result. Some illnesses can, however, lead to a specific physical disability, for example, one related to hearing or sight. In these cases it is important that the employer does not assume the employee is unable to continue duties because of the disability. Rather, the employer can investigate ways in which the working environment can be adapted and equipped to overcome barriers to the employee continuing work as usual.

There are numerous types of equipment and adaptations which can be made to most working environments to ensure that people with physical disabilities are able to work on an equal basis with others. There are also many organisations which can advise the employer as to how the workplace can be adapted and the financial help which is available to achieve this. The Royal National Institute for the Blind (RNIB) and the Royal National Institute for the Deaf (RNID) are examples of organisations which can provide sources of guidance.

There may be some occasions when an employer thinks that their organisation is not able to or cannot afford to keep a person employed because they have a health problem or disability. There are, however, a number of schemes which can provide outside help, including financial help, for employers. The Access to Work scheme is an example of a government-run scheme which can give financial help.

Access to Work

The Access to Work (ATW) scheme is based at job centres and is administered by the Placement, Assessment and Counselling (PAC) teams. The teams employ Disability Employment Advisers who are specialists on disability. There are also technical officers who can advise about equipment and adaptations which can be acquired under the ATW scheme. The type of help given by the scheme includes:

adaptations to premises or equipment; special aids and equipment for a disabled person; help with the costs of employing a personal reader for a person who has a visual impairment; and various other ways of providing financial support for employing someone with a disability. The ATW scheme does not necessarily pay all of the costs incurred by the employer, but does pay a substantial proportion.

Supervision and Monitoring

Section 6 (3) (l) providing supervision

When an agreement has been made between the employer and an employee who is affected by illness about the way in which work is to be continued, it is important to set up mechanisms to ensure these working practices are regularly reviewed.

Any targets set, for example, should be supervised and monitored regularly with the employee to ensure that they are still appropriate and achievable. The work capacity of people with long-term or frequent intermittent illnesses may vary considerably over time. The regular monitoring of targets can ensure that alternative agreements for ways of working can be reached, if an existing method proves inappropriate. This is one way of increasing the potential for meeting targets overall.

Conclusion

This chapter has looked at the implications of the DDA in relation to HIV. Ideas have been given for how organisations could comply with the Act by adapting or modifying workplace conditions or arrangements for people with HIV related illnesses. In the previous chapter we looked at how, in the absence of specific legislation, general laws could be applied to people who are HIV positive and asymptomatic.

Out of this discussion two main areas can be identified for policy. The first is that all employers will want to develop policy and procedures which ensure that they comply with all aspects of the law. Policy and procedures on long-term and intermittent illness, for example, could be developed to incorporate HIV related illness.

The second policy area is employment protection for all people affected by HIV. Within employment law there are clear gaps in the protection afforded to people who are HIV positive and asymptomatic. The DDA does give protection to such people but with a number of qualifications to how and when the protection is afforded. Forward thinking organisations will, therefore, want to ensure that their policies and procedures give people with HIV the same employment protection as any other employees – regardless of whether employment law does or does not require it.

4 Confidentiality

Introduction

This Chapter looks at the factors which employers should consider when addressing the issue of confidentiality in relation to HIV. The chapter starts by explaining the ethical and legal obligations to maintain confidential information about HIV and goes on to give principles and policy points which can be adopted by all employers regardless of their size or type. The chapter then discusses areas which will only be relevant to particular types of organisations, that is, those in the statutory and independent sectors providing services related to health and community care. At the end of the chapter, an excerpt from the guidelines on confidentiality by the General Medical Council (GMC) is reproduced for reference.

HIV and Confidentiality in Context

Imagine going to get the results of an HIV test in any small city or town in Britain. You would probably come home full of feelings and emotion and a desperate need to talk to somebody. But who do you tell? How do you know if a friend or family member will keep a confidence? Can you tell your doctor or dentist? Who might they tell – and is there anyone they *have* to tell? If word gets out – in your neighbourhood, at local shops, at your job – how will it affect your life, including specific matters like insurance cover, job security, parenting and healthcare?

In the case of HIV, an unwarranted fear and hatred of some groups (gay men, for example) can combine to produce real harm or danger to people with HIV when their identities are inadvertently or deliberately revealed. Since people in Britain became aware of HIV and AIDS in the early 1980s there have been many examples of discrimination not only against people who are HIV positive but also against people who are assumed to be, especially gay men. Examples include being refused or dismissed from employment; being victimised in their neighbourhood by taunting, threats and verbal harassment; and being the target of physical violence in many different situations.

The responsibility to protect confidentiality of people who are HIV positive should not therefore only relate to legal obligations but to ethical ones as well. Any organisation providing services to the public and any organisation employing staff should have a particularly compelling duty in this regard. We begin by looking at the legal situation.

Employment Law and Confidentiality

In common law there is a duty to keep information confidential if it was given in trust and if that information is not generally known. However, because there is no right to privacy in British law, it is difficult to mount cases against a breach of confidentiality.

Under employment law, the contract of employment has within it an implied duty of 'mutual trust and confidence' for both employer and employee. The duty of trust and confidence includes a duty for both employer and employee not to disclose confidential information obtained in the course of employment.

The case of *X* v. *Y and another* in 1987 gives legal backing to the claim that an employee would be in breach of confidence if they disclosed the names of anyone who was HIV positive. Southam and Howard, 'AIDS and Employment Law' describe the case as follows:

> ... the Queen's Bench Division of the High Court held that the names of anyone suffering from AIDS should remain confidential. A national newspaper was restrained

> from publishing the names of two doctors still practising medicine who were being treated at the hospital for AIDS. The High Court ruled that the public and patients were entitled to expect that hospital records be kept confidential and 'it was not for any individual to take it upon himself or herself to breach that confidence'.[1]

It seems clear from this case that any employer or employee who disclosed information about a person's HIV status without the individual's consent would be considered to have breached the duty of confidence to the individual concerned. The only exception to this rule is if it could be claimed that it was in the public interest for others to know – this is a standard defence against breach of confidence claims. Some organisations, especially those dealing with medical issues, may need to seek specialised legal advice about areas where there is conflict between the individual's right to confidence and 'the public interest'.

The Data Protection Act 1984 gives extra weight to confidentiality, although these laws relate only to information recorded on equipment. HIV is not specifically mentioned in the Act but the devastating effect that breach of confidentiality can have in relation to HIV means that employers should act scrupulously to ensure that they do comply with the Act.

Laws on confidentiality and HIV are further strengthened in Health Authorities by the National Health Service (Venereal Diseases) Regulations 1974, Section 1, 1974.9. The regulations place a duty on Health Authorities to maintain the confidentiality of any information obtained by their officers which could identify a person being treated for a sexually transmitted disease. It is, of course, permissible for confidential information to be shared between medical practitioners and other relevant staff if it is relevant to the treatment of the individual. Local Authorities are also bound by this duty.

Maintaining Confidentiality

In order to comply with their duty of confidence, employers need to ensure that they have, and supervise compliance with, effective procedures to keep confidential any records which may contain information on an employee's HIV status. It is clearly in the employers' interests to have clear policy and practice on confidentiality.

Even when disclosure without consent is justified, it should only be to those who have a real need to know the information. Disclosure should be on the basis that the information is strictly confidential and should not be further disclosed.

Because disclosure of a person's HIV status may have serious consequences, the employer would probably be justified in treating such a disclosure as a serious disciplinary offence.

Is Information about HIV any Different from Other Information?

Information concerning HIV is different from other information in some respects. The differences are that the need for confidentiality about HIV information is heightened, not in a legal sense, but because public fear about HIV is still very high. Also, there are sometimes strong feelings among staff, and sometimes clients, about the 'right to know' versus confidentiality.

Dealing with Confidentiality in the Workplace

A few general principles can be used to inform discussion about any specific issues which arise in relation to confidentiality. These are as follows:

1. Organisations should assume that all staff and clients are already HIV positive in order to put the issue in perspective.

2. Organisations should actively safeguard and protect confidentiality about the HIV status of all staff and clients.

3. When the HIV status of a staff member or client is known, either through recorded information or verbally, the indisputable 'need to know' is the criterion for disclosure. What constitutes such need should be determined beforehand through standards and rules.

4. Organisations should not pressure any employee or client to reveal their HIV status. The truth is that most organisations providing services to clients do not need to know the clients' HIV status in order to provide the services available.

5. Organisations should provide education to all staff, and as appropriate, to clients about basic issues and policy relating to confidentiality, so that inadvertent breaches can be avoided.

Some organisations do not deal with information about individual clients and many more would not be in a position to have information which could possibly include a client's HIV status: in these types of organisations it is still crucial to have policy which addresses the issue of confidentiality for staff.

Essential Elements for Policies on Confidentiality

Every organisation, regardless of its types of clients or customers, can adopt the following elements, based on the above principles, into a confidentiality policy.

- Confidentiality should be ensured for all personal and medical information, including an employee's HIV status.

- Should the fact become known that an employee or user of the organisation has the virus, then strict confidentiality will be maintained.

- Only those people with a genuine reason to know that a person has HIV will be informed. No one will be informed without the written consent of the person affected by HIV.

- An employee with HIV whose status is known, should be protected from discrimination, and this is most likely to be achieved through participatory education in the workplace.

- Deliberate breaches of confidentiality will be considered a disciplinary offence.

For organisations that do deal with clients or residents it is important that the organisation's policy on confidentiality does cover information from and about clients. For organisations that have a remit to provide welfare, social or medical services of any kind to clients, it is essential to have comprehensive confidentiality policies.

The following discussion of policy questions and recommendations will be useful for organisations that deal with welfare, social or medical issues in relation to clients. The guidelines will also be useful for organisations which provide either permanent or temporary accommodation for residents.

Policy Questions and Recommendations

1. Should a new client's or resident's HIV status be requested?

If the basic assumption is made that all staff and clients are currently infected, then requesting clients to reveal their HIV status (if known) seems counterproductive. Furthermore, it raises the thorny question of how to record or manage the information acquired through such a question. Finally, it may only encourage clients to lie, especially when they are new to an organisation and have not yet developed a level of trust that makes honesty possible. Generally, questions about whether or not the client has taken the HIV antibody test, or what the client's (known) status might be, need not be asked at all during the admission process.

2. Who needs to know a client's or resident's HIV status?

When a client or resident reveals their status to staff in an organisation it may seem logical to assume that other staff may need to know. But 'need to know' has always been an uncertain principle, open to varying interpretation.

The first answer is that any time a staff member intends to reveal a client's or resident's HIV status to other staff, they should inform the client or resident and obtain their consent in writing beforehand, letting him or her know who is being informed and why. Not only is this courtesy, it is also sound practice.

Beyond that, no definitive answer is possible. However, organisations should consider the following when determining who among staff (and if appropriate volunteers) 'needs to know':

- The client's or resident's right to privacy.
- The organisation's possible liability.
- The continuity of care, especially medical care.
- The potential for discrimination against the individual, both within and outside of the organisation.
- The extent to which the organisation's staff are trained and knowledgeable about HIV issues.

Such guidelines should be established before questions of 'need to know' arise in actual practice.

3. *Should clients or residents be expected to reveal results if they are tested during the course of treatment?*

The client or resident should not be expected to disclose to everybody; most people will carefully consider who needs to know and who does not, who is 'safe' to tell and who is not (including staff), and make self-disclosure decisions accordingly. As for the staff, there may be considerable benefit to the client or resident in letting them know that 'it's up to you, but if you want to disclose your results, we may be of some help'.

4. Is the organisation responsible if another client or resident breaks confidentiality about a client's or resident's antibody status?

Organisations dealing with clients or residents for social and medical treatment will be well aware that even when staff uphold confidential obligations, clients or residents will often disclose personal information to each other, sometimes with unfortunate consequences. There have been a few cases, for example, of a resident disclosing their HIV status to another resident in the same project, in strict confidence, only to find the vow of secrecy broken.

Legally, the organisation cannot usually be held to be vicariously liable if a client or resident has divulged confidential information about another client or resident. If, however, a client or resident has obtained information about another because the organisation's records and information have not been securely stored, then the organisation may be shown to be liable. Although the organisation may not be legally liable for a breach of confidence between clients or residents, it is good practice to take practical measures to try to stop this happening.

First, when a client or resident reports that they are HIV positive to a staff member, they should receive specific counselling and support guidance about who to inform and who it might be best not to inform. Clients and residents should be assisted in thinking through, with careful consideration of possible consequences, their own self-disclosure plan or strategy. Second, clients, residents and staff should all receive, as part of their comprehensive HIV education, specific information on HIV confidentiality and information about the organisation's confidentiality policy. In addition, clients and residents should be advised of the importance of honouring the HIV related confidence of a friend or acquaintance.

5. If the organisation maintains files that identify a client's or resident's HIV status and the client or resident is transferred to another agency, should the information identifying HIV status also be transferred?

The most appropriate strategy is to allow the client or resident to reveal her or his antibody status to others as she or he deems fitting and useful. File transfer of information may undermine that approach. It will usually be preferable to keep such information out of individual files in the first place. In this way, organisations can avoid the dilemma of the transfer of sensitive information and serve the client's or resident's best interests at the same time.

Some organisations may, of course, be dealing with a client or resident because they have problems related to HIV. Likewise, a transfer or referral to another agency may specifically be about an HIV related issue. In these cases, it is important first to discuss the transfer or referral with the client or resident and preferably to have written permission for disclosure from them. Second, the principle of 'need to know' is of paramount importance when giving information to another organisation and agreements about confidentiality should be secured between agencies.

Medical Guidelines on Confidentiality

The following guidelines have been issued by the General Medical Council about confidentiality for doctors and health-care workers in relation to HIV.

> Doctors are familiar with the need to make judgements about whether to disclose confidential information in particular circumstances, and the need to justify their action where such a disclosure is made. The GMC believes that, where HIV infection or AIDS has been diagnosed, any difficulties concerning confidentiality which arise will usually be overcome if doctors are prepared to discuss openly and honestly with patients the implications of their condition, the need to secure the safety of others, and the importance for continuing medical care of ensuring that those who will be involved need to know the nature of their condition and the particular needs which they will have. The GMC takes the view that any doctor who discovers that a patient is

HIV positive or suffering from AIDS has a duty to discuss these matters fully with the patient.

Informing other healthcare professionals

When a patient is seen by a specialist who diagnoses HIV infection or AIDS and a general practitioner is or may become involved in that patient's care, then the specialist should explain to the patient that the general practitioner cannot be expected to provide adequate clinical management and care without full knowledge of the patient's condition. The GMC believes that the majority of such patients will readily be persuaded of the need for their general practitioners to be informed of the diagnosis.

If the patient refuses consent for the general practitioner to be told, then the doctor has two sets of obligations to consider: obligations to the patient to maintain confidence, and obligations to other carers whose own health may be put unnecessarily at risk. In such circumstances the patient should be counselled about the difficulties which his or her condition are likely to pose for the team responsible for providing continuing healthcare and about the likely consequences for the standard of care which can be provided in the future. If, having considered the matter carefully in the light of such counselling, the patient still refuses to allow the general practitioner to be informed, then the patient's request for privacy should be respected. The only exception to that general principle arises where the doctor judges that the failure to disclose would put the health of any of the healthcare team at serious risk. The GMC believes that, in such a situation, it would not be improper to disclose such information as the person needs to know. The need for such a decision is, in present circumstances, likely to arise only rarely, but if it is made the doctor must be able to justify his or her actions.

Similar principles apply to the sharing of confidential information between specialists or with other healthcare professionals such as nurses, laboratory technicians and dentists. All persons receiving such information must, of course, consider themselves under the same general obligation of confidentiality as the doctor principally responsible for the patient's care.

Informing the patient's spouse or other sexual partner

Questions of conflicting obligations also arise when a doctor is faced with deciding whether the fact that a patient is HIV positive or suffering from AIDS should be disclosed to a third party, other than another health professional, without the consent of the patient. The GMC has reached the view that there are grounds for disclosure only where there is a serious and identifiable risk to a specific individual who, if not so informed, would be exposed to infection. Therefore, when a person is found to be infected in this way, the doctor must discuss with the patient the question of informing a spouse or other sexual partner. The GMC believes that most patients will agree to disclosure in these circumstances, but where such consent is withheld the doctor may consider it his duty to seek to ensure that any sexual partner is informed, in order to safeguard such persons from infection.[2]

5 The HIV Antibody Test

In Chapter 2, 'HIV and Employment Law', the legal situation is described for employers asking employees to take an HIV antibody test. This chapter explores some of the wider employment issues which arise in relation to this test.

The chapter starts with general information, principles and guidelines for all organisations. The latter part of the chapter gives more specific guidelines for organisations or departments in the statutory and independent sectors that provide services related to health and community care.

About the HIV Antibody Test

When people speak of 'the HIV test', they are usually referring to two specific test procedures which determine the presence or absence of the HIV antibody. These tests are the ELISA (Enzyme-linked Immunosorbent Assay) and the Western Blot. In the UK the ELISA is the most commonly used and thought by many to be the more reliable. The tests are performed by taking a sample of blood or saliva.

Because the ELISA has been known to produce false positive results on some occasions, either the Western Blot or another ELISA test is generally used to 'double check' a positive ELISA test result.

Although taking an HIV antibody test is relatively simple and straightforward, there are many considerations related to testing which make the whole reality of testing much more complex.

Basic Principles for Policy

There are a few essential principles that should govern our approach to, and conclusions about, HIV antibody testing. These principles can be used by any organisation to formulate policy in relation to HIV testing and the workplace.

1. No one should be forced to take the test against his or her will without incontestable cause and consent. Of course, such a clause can be widely interpreted but the basic ethic is pre-eminent. Mandatory testing, without consent, is an invasion of a person's very being and cannot be required unless there is some other value, more compelling, that overrules it.

2. No one should be tested unless true, informed consent has first been given. A signature on a form that few take time to read may cover an organisation for contractual or legal reasons. But true, informed consent insists that individuals being tested know what the test is, how it works, what it does and does not do and the personal, social and financial (for example, insurance) consequences of positive and negative results.

3. Testing should not be used as a screening device for employment or services. Not only is it an inaccurate predictor of who is in fact positive at any one time, it also serves no purpose and may be illegal in certain circumstances.

4. In order to make informed decisions about being tested, individuals have the right to all available information about testing, including the range of opinions about the advantages and disadvantages of testing. The implication for those giving advice about being tested is clear: we are here to provide, or assist in the provision of, all the facts and viewpoints we have at our disposal, perhaps even those that ran counter to our personal views. This approach avoids the possibility of people feeling that they have been coerced into being tested.

Reasons for Not Requiring Workplace Testing

1. Testing employees cannot give an employer reliable information about an employee's HIV status. There is a 'window period' between being infected with HIV and producing antibodies to the virus. The 'window period' can be up to six months and, in rare cases, even longer. Therefore, an employee who has been infected with HIV could still show negative on an antibody test.

2. Testing all employees or new recruits for HIV is expensive. In addition, for a company to have more reliable results about HIV, it would have to test employees regularly: about every three to six months. Regular testing of all employees would be extremely expensive.

3. The mere presence of HIV tells the employer nothing about the individual's capacity to do a particular job.

4. People who are HIV positive may live more than twenty years without developing any related illnesses. It is possible that some people with HIV may never develop any related illnesses. Therefore, if the purpose of testing employees is to 'sift-out' employees who may become ill, the efficiency of this approach is extremely doubtful.

5. Requiring employees to be tested may be open to legal challenges (see Chapter 2).

6. A positive result to a test may have a devastating effect on the individual.

There are relatively few organisations that do insist on HIV testing. However, those that do include large companies: a number of airlines, following the example of British Airways, have introduced testing for cabin staff.

The British Government, the World Health Organisation, the International Labour Organisation and the Council of Europe are amongst many who have stated clearly that there are no grounds for testing people for HIV either pre-employment or in employment. However, it would seem that until a law is passed to forbid such discriminatory practices then certain companies will continue to ignore advice.

Is it Ever Reasonable to Ask Employees to be Tested?

There are some areas where employers have argued that there is a genuine need for employees to be tested: one which is not related to prejudice or undue caution about HIV. These are as follows.

1. Working Abroad

There are some occupations where an employee may be required to work in countries which have mandatory HIV antibody testing for anyone working there: a positive result would be a bar to working in that country. In such cases, it seems reasonable that the employee who is required to work in these countries should be encouraged to be tested at a Genito-Urinary Medicine (GUM) clinic before they leave the UK. The advantage of being tested at a GUM is that pre- and post-test counselling is given in order to prepare and help a person with the results of the test. This is much preferable to suddenly finding out you are HIV positive from the results of testing by immigration authorities.

Some qualifying points are needed, however, before asking employees to be tested to work abroad.

1. It should have been made clear to the employee at recruitment that they may be required to work in countries which have mandatory HIV testing.

2. Working in such countries should be a genuine requirement of the job: seconding employees to certain countries should not be used as an excuse to force employees to be tested. If it is not a genuine requirement the employer may be open to claims of 'constructive dismissal'.

3. If an employee does not want to be tested, the employer should explore all other possibilities for working arrangements. For example, it may be that the employer sends many employees to many different countries, only some of which require testing. In such situations, it could be policy that only those employees who undertake voluntary testing are sent to countries with mandatory testing requirements.

2. Sparse Conditions

A survey by the Labour Research Department[1] based on questionnaires filled in by trade union branch secretaries identified only one employer – out of 400 workplaces – who did pre-employment testing. The employer was the National Environment Research Council (NERC), which conducts research into all aspects of the environment. It is only a very specific group of workers who are tested, that is approximately 100 staff who set out on the British Antarctic Survey (BAS) each year. The tests are part of a pre-employment health check and those employed are mostly contract staff who are recruited annually. Counselling is offered both before and after testing. The NERC emphasise the particular context in which HIV testing takes place, that being:

> the extreme conditions in which staff have to work, the sparse medical facilities and the possibility that staff may have to provide blood for use in transfusions for their colleagues.[2]

Although the arguments set out by the NERC are reasonable in these specific circumstances, it should be stressed that the circumstances described by the NERC are quite unique.

Employment in Healthcare

In the 1980s, there was considerable debate as to whether all healthcare workers should be tested for HIV antibodies as a condition of service. Occasionally, the debate is resurrected today when alarmist press reports cause fear among the public.

Those within the profession generally recognise that the risk of transmission of HIV from practitioner to patient is extremely small; the risk is usually only associated with the use of invasive surgery techniques.

The approach taken by the General Medical Council (GMC) in relation to doctors and other health workers puts the debate into perspective by stressing personal responsibility and ethical considerations. GMC guidelines do not suggest forcing anyone to be tested against their will. It is stressed, however, that doctors and other health workers with HIV infection are ethically obliged to seek professional advice on whether or not they need to limit or modify their practice to protect their patients. GMC guidance, 'HIV and AIDS: the ethical considerations', states:

> ... it is imperative, both in the public interest and on ethical grounds, that any doctor who thinks they may have been infected with HIV should seek appropriate diagnostic testing and counselling and, if found to be infected, have regular medical supervision.
>
> Doctors who are HIV positive should also seek specialist advice on the extent to which they should limit their practice in order to protect their patients. Such advice will usually be obtained from a consultant in occupational health, who may in turn seek guidance, on an anonymous basis, from the UK Advisory Panel of the Expert Advisory Group on AIDS. Doctors must act upon that advice which, in some circumstances, would include a requirement not to practise or to limit their practice in certain ways. No doctor should continue in clinical practice merely on the basis of their own assessment of the risks to patients ...
>
> It is unethical for doctors who know or believe themselves to be infected with HIV to put patients at risk by failing to seek appropriate counselling or by failing to act upon it when given. Such behaviour may result in

proceedings by the GMC which could lead to the restriction or removal of a doctor's registration if this were necessary to protect patients' or the doctor's own health.[3]

The guidelines make it clear that the risk of a doctor who is HIV positive endangering a patient is 'very small'. When the 1995 edition of the guidelines was published, there was only one known case in the whole world of a healthcare worker transmitting HIV to patients: in the course of dental treatment. Therefore, although healthcare professionals should seek the prescribed specialist advice, in the vast majority of cases, no limitation is needed and there is no reason or obligation to inform the employer.

Some Questions to Consider about Testing

In organisations which have well-developed personnel and welfare services for employees, and for organisations which give advice to clients on health and welfare issues, there may be occasions when advice is sought about whether or not an HIV antibody test should be taken. In these situations it is always advisable to refer people to appropriately trained, professional HIV advisers. Some indicators can be given, however, as to the type of questions the individual should ask themselves before being tested. These are:

- Do I know what the test is, and what it does and does not do?
- Are my reasons for being tested logical and well reasoned?
- Have I considered what I will do if the test results are positive? Negative?
- Am I aware that no matter how the test result turns out, the real focus is behaviour and possible change?
- Am I aware of the difference between being tested at a GUM and being testing privately?

- Do I need to be tested immediately, do I need more information, or do I need to wait a while?

- If I decide to be tested, is there a 'support person' who can help me through the process?

Some Pros and Cons of Being Tested

On the one hand ...

- While to date, there is no way of reversing HIV infection, many in the medical profession believe that early determination of seropositivity can lead to medical interventions that may help to stem the replication of the virus.

- Early detection of HIV can lead to lifestyle and behaviour changes that may support the maintenance of long-term health and well-being.

- For some, being tested may help awareness about the importance of behaviour change that will reduce the risk of infecting others or becoming infected.

- For others, there is considerable anxiety surrounding the possibility of HIV infection, and the only way that anxiety is relieved is by being tested.

- The results of the HIV antibody test can assist individuals in their personal decision-making about childbearing, family planning, relationships and other matters.

- Finally, early detection of HIV can enable early notification of the person's sexual or intravenous drug partners who may be at risk of HIV infection.

On the other hand ...

- Some people have heard a lot about the test, but actually know very little about it. Some have come to believe that the test 'does something' that will protect them from infection. In fact, the only thing the test 'does' is indicate the presence or otherwise of the HIV antibody.

- Some have used the test as a way to give themselves a 'clean bill of health', so that they can return to previous behaviours without concern.

- Some people may not be psychologically or emotionally prepared to hear that they are HIV positive. Unprepared individuals are vulnerable to a wide range of emotional responses ranging from denial to utter despair.

- Some people might choose to have the test because they have heard repeated recommendations from others to do so. But being tested is a uniquely personal thing; such blanket recommendations are not germane to the individual and his or her situation.

- Some new couples are being tested simultaneously so that they do not have to use condoms or other precautions when having sex. But to be truly effective, such a strategy has to take into account the six-month window period, and places considerable trust in ongoing sexual and needle-sharing monogamy.

6 HIV Related Discrimination In Context

Introduction

Since the beginning of the HIV epidemic, the virus has been associated with individuals or classes of people who have already suffered rejection, discrimination and prejudice. In the UK, HIV and AIDS have affected gay men more than heterosexuals and black and ethnic minority heterosexual people proportionally more than white heterosexual people.[1] Rates of HIV infection are proportionally higher among intravenous drug users, and sex workers (prostitutes) are often assumed to have higher rates of HIV than the rest of the population. Globally, people who are poor are more likely to become HIV infected than the more affluent. In many counties the poor have less access to healthcare if they become ill.

These facts have, unfortunately, added fuel to discrimination. Faced with the enormity of HIV, it seems some people will look to someone else to blame. In view of this, it is essential that organisations which aim to ensure that people with HIV are treated fairly, make certain that groups of people affected are also given protection.

People with HIV have faced discrimination in the areas of employment, housing, finance and insurance, immigration, prisons, by the police and the courts. This chapter looks at some of the many ways in which people with HIV have experienced discrimination. Many of the examples given illustrate why it is so important for the policy areas identified in this book – such as testing, confidentiality, and comprehensive non-discrimination strategies – to be dealt with effectively in any organisation.

The chapter starts with some examples of HIV related employment discrimination. However, the chapter goes on to show that discrimination on the grounds of HIV is rarely isolated from other forms of discrimination. In many cases, HIV has compounded problems for people who already face discrimination because of their sex, race, sexuality, and so forth. Whilst recognising that all forms of discrimination are equally important, the second half of the chapter concentrates mainly on discrimination on the grounds of sexuality rather than other forms of discrimination. This is because the nature and extent of discrimination against lesbians and gay men is not widely documented. It is therefore necessary to give more detail here about sexuality than about areas on which much has already been written. For example, there is much research which shows indisputably that, although race and sex discrimination are illegal, both are still highly prevalent in the UK. The Equal Opportunities Commission (EOC) and the Commission for Racial Equality (CRE) both produce a range of publications which highlight discrimination in many areas of life, including employment.

HIV Discrimination in Employment

There are a number of reports which document the type of discrimination experienced by people who are affected by HIV. Some of these reports are quoted below to illustrate just some of the ways in which HIV related discrimination has manifested itself in work related situations. The first two examples below are reported in 'Unequal Opportunities' (1994), a report from the National Association of Citizen's Advice Bureaux (NACAB). The report uses evidence from actual cases dealt with by local Citizen's Advice Bureaux (CABx). The first is a typical example of the type of harassment people have faced because of HIV.

> A CAB in East Sussex reported a client who had been employed as an assistant manager in a shop. His partner had an AIDS-related illness, and when this become known to his colleagues, the client experienced harass-

ment. Colleagues left the dining room when he came in to eat, he was kept away from customers, and was required to wash the toilet with bleach after he had used it. He was subsequently dismissed for bad time keeping.[2]

The second example illustrates how a woman was forced to have an HIV test or risk losing her job.

A CAB in Dorset reported a client who had worked part time in a nursing home for six months. The employer received an anonymous phone call stating that the client was HIV positive, and then suspended the client without pay until she submitted a negative HIV test result.[3]

In 1997, three years after the above report was written, NACAB are continuing to receive reports from local CABx about problems and discrimination experienced by clients in relation to HIV and employment.

In the past, people with HIV have been sacked purely because they are perceived to be or are HIV positive. Immunity, a legal centre for people affected by HIV, gives the following example in their 1994–95 Annual Report.

An HIV positive man working in a large hospital disclosed his HIV status to his employers. Despite at first being offered redeployment, he was soon threatened with dismissal and came to Immunity for advice. We wrote to the employers pointing out the Government's guidelines on dealing with infected healthcare workers and also wrote to the Department of Health for guidance on whether it was necessary for him to be redeployed. Despite this letter, he was not redeployed and was later sacked for being 'incapable of performing his job'.[4]

Lesbian and Gay Employment Rights (LAGER), an advice and information agency for lesbians and gay men with work related problems, has dealt with hundreds of examples of gay men who have had problems at work related to HIV. In the following example from LAGER, the employee was effectively forced to resign but did not take legal action because he was unlikely to be awarded more money at an industrial tribunal than his employers offered to give him to leave.

> Andrew worked for a small private firm in the service industry. His work involved day-to-day contact with the public. During his employment, he developed Kaposi's sarcoma, a type of skin cancer associated with HIV, which spread to his face. His employers said that they were worried that the public he dealt with might be upset if they saw his face and they offered Andrew a sum of money to leave.[5]

Although all of the above exemplify typical problems which people who are or are suspected to be HIV positive have had, the next sections try to put HIV discrimination in context with other forms of discrimination.

HIV and Sexism

As with other forms of discrimination, it is sometimes difficult to know whether discrimination has occurred against an HIV positive woman because of her sex, her race or because of her HIV status. Sometimes all three apply. There is a lack of information generally about the effect of HIV on women. Jonathan Glasson remarks:

> The portrayal of HIV as something which only concerns certain 'high risk groups' has led to a damaging failure to focus on the specific experiences and problems of women. There is a serious lack of data showing the impact of HIV on women.[6]

Much of the attention given to women and HIV has focused on their roles as 'vectors of transmission' – sex workers (prostitutes) who could infect men, pregnant women who could infect children – rather than the issues and needs of HIV infected women themselves. Not enough attention has been paid to women who are HIV positive and have dependants. An HIV infected mother, for example, may find it more difficult to maintain employment or access HIV services due to lack of childcare resources.

One of the few organisations to respond to and investigate the problems facing women with HIV infection is the voluntary organisation, Positively Women. From 1992 to 1994, Positively Women carried out the first piece of community based HIV research into the needs of HIV positive women in the UK. Interviews were carried out with 75 HIV positive women from a broad range of cultural backgrounds.[7]

The findings of the research, published in the report 'Women Like Us', found that over half of the women interviewed (53.3%) had experienced some form of discrimination because of their HIV status. Various problems and discrimination were reported, including being tested for HIV without their consent; feeling pressured not to become pregnant or to have an abortion; a lack of home care and child minding support and problems with housing, healthcare and social services.

All of these problems can cause additional difficulties for women who are trying to maintain jobs or find employment.

HIV and Racism

No reasonable person would argue that racism is no longer with us, or that it does not affect all areas of life. Racism, like homophobia, has been fuelled by 'AIDSphobia'. The report 'Luxury or Necessity?' illustrates this point.

> A black straight man was housed in a specialist scheme for people with HIV. He suffered harassment when the nature of the block became known. He was verbally abused about both his HIV status and his race, received hate mail, and had graffiti daubed on his house.[8]

The research by Positively Women found that nearly one in five women had been tested without their consent. All of those tested without consent between 1988 and the time of the survey were African women. Furthermore, African women tested in this period were less likely to have received pre-test counselling.[9]

The following account from 'Luxury or Necessity?' shows a disturbing case of testing without consent and a possible serious breach of confidentiality.

> An African immigrant, whose English was poor, was tested without their understanding. When they went back for their result, they saw 'AIDS' on the front of the folder. No one in the hospital could speak their language and a translator had not been arranged. In the end, the nurses sought out the only other person in the hospital who could speak the language and asked them to tell the immigrant that 'They have AIDS'. This person was the cleaner.[10]

In addition to the more blatant forms of discrimination, there are other ways in which black people with HIV have often felt that services and organisations have not responded well to their cultural realities and needs. A lot of the early HIV material proved to be culturally insensitive: for example, safer sex information was translated literally from English to another language without exploring cultural meanings behind the actual words and phrases used.

As in the case of gay men, black people, especially people from Africa, have often been assumed to be HIV infected, simply because of their identity. For black gay men this assumption has been made from both angles.

Lesbians and Gay Men

Background: HIV and Homophobia

Much of the animosity that has surfaced around the issue of HIV has been directed at gay men, bisexuals and sometimes lesbians too. First a few definitions are in order. A 'gay man' refers to a man who experiences the human need for warmth, affection and love from persons of the same gender; sometimes this includes sexual contact. A 'lesbian' is a woman who experiences the need for warmth, affection and love from persons of the same gender; sometimes this includes sexual contact. A 'bisexual' is a person who experiences the need for warmth, affection and love from persons of either gender; sometimes this includes sexual contact. The animosity towards these groups of people is commonly referred to as *homophobia*.

Homophobia is defined as an irrational fear or dread of homosexuality or homosexuals, or an inordinate fear of intimate relationships with others of the same gender. What makes homophobia a social problem rather than a personal attitude, is that those fears are reinforced by law and culture: in this sense, homophobia is institutionalised.

Under British law, it is still not illegal to discriminate against a lesbian or a gay man in employment, housing, family relationships and many other areas of life.

Some areas of British law actively discriminate against lesbians and gay men. For example, the 1956 Sexual Offences Act and the 1967 Sexual Offences Act both contain laws which discriminate against gay men: there is an unequal age of consent for gay men and a number of offences that gay men can be charged with that would not be considered crimes if the acts were performed by members of the opposite sex.

In the armed forces contact between members of the same sex, either male or female, has been decriminalised. However, contact is still forbidden whether the person is on or off duty or on leave. Anyone discovered to be lesbian or gay in the armed forces will be automatically discharged (at the time of writing this point is being challenged via the European courts).

Types of Discrimination

A study by Social and Community Planning Research (SCPR), an independent research institute, set out to look at the nature of discrimination against lesbians and gay men in Britain today. The survey draws on the experiences of 116 lesbians and gay men. The study also includes responses from 619 heterosexuals who are asked to give views about lesbians and gay men and their perceptions of whether or not discrimination occurs. The survey reports high levels of discrimination in many areas of life, including employment.

The survey respondents were asked about a number of possible ways in which they might personally have experienced discrimination. These covered experiences related to work, renting accommodation, obtaining insurance, and personally abusive incidents. Approximately half had experienced at least one of the forms of discrimination listed.[11]

Attitudes towards HIV and AIDS were explicitly linked by some of the respondents to the levels of discrimination.

> " I think with AIDS it's getting worse because people automatically say homosexuals have brought this disease on to everybody. But I think when you have pop bands doing really good things like when Freddie Mercury died and things like that. It's like, oh, he was a hero, you know, it sort of smoothed the path out a bit and everything was all right for a while and then it all starts up again. (Lesbian, 20s, Midlands town)[12]

> " Well for every step forward the gay community makes in teaching people about HIV and AIDS there's the trashy tabloid press taking two steps back, so I suppose AIDS does make a difference because people do tend to believe what they read. (Gay man, 20s, SE town)[13]

Employment Discrimination

Employment is a major area where lesbians and gay men have suffered discrimination because of their sexuality. As with other forms of discrimination it is often difficult to know whether a gay man has been discriminated against for his sexuality or his perceived HIV status. Again, both may be the case. It is worth noting that the HIV related tribunal cases referred to in Chapter 2 all involve gay men who were discriminated against because of their perceived, rather than known, HIV status.

Even in the absence of HIV, lesbians and gay men have been refused jobs and promotion and have been dismissed because of their sexuality. Harassment of lesbians and gay men is not uncommon and such harassment can include both verbal and physical abuse.

In November 1996 the Institute of Personnel and Development (IPD) carried out qualitative interviews with recruitment consultants, workers and campaign groups around the UK to see whether they felt that some groups of people were more likely to encounter discrimination from employers when seeking work. Generally, the recruitment consultants interviewed did not think that lesbians and gay men suffered discrimination in employment. The examples given in the IPD report from workers, however, illustrate that harassment is still a problem for lesbians and gay men. In addition, many of the old stereotypes about lesbians and gay men – as child molesters, as sexual predators, and so on – still exist today. The example below is from Andrew who works for a large distribution company based in West Lothian.

> “ I've been working as a forklift driver for the company for the last six months. I don't flaunt being gay, but I don't cover it either. There's a lot of people in work who don't like me for that, especially among the floor staff. The worst thing was being accused of being a child abuser. It only took one person to say that, and when he did, I had to go to one of the supervisors to say, 'Get this guy pulled aside else I'm going to do something about it myself.' He did get pulled aside, but obviously mud sticks.
>
> On a long shift they'll all start laughing and joking about me: 'Do you fancy this guy?' If I try and share the joke, and say, 'Oh aye, you're alright', they'll accuse me of sexual harassment, saying 'I'm going upstairs to management for a word about this.' I'm getting called names, and a lot of people in the building won't even speak to me because they think I'm a child abuser. There's people with a reputation for being hard nuts here, and as they're getting wind of this child abuse stuff, it's creating hassle for me.[14]

In a similar vein, another example given in the IPD report illustrates that the stereotype of lesbians both as 'butch' on the one hand, but only needing sex with a man to put 'to put them right' on the other hand, is still very much alive. Elise works for a Manchester-based accountancy firm.

> " I've been with the company for two years doing a very sober job. For the first 18 months, nobody, but nobody, knew that I was a lesbian. Then somebody who remembered my wilder days at university moved to the company. I don't think that she was being malicious, but word seeped out around the building. One morning, one of my immediate superiors brushed past me in the hall and said in a really nasty tone of voice, 'I hear you're too butch to pull a man, Elise.' Usually, I'd have come back with a put-down, but he was my boss. I just had to take it.
>
> Since then, he's been on a one-man crusade to make my life miserable. It's 'Got your bull-dyke knickers on today, Elise?' and, 'Fancy a quick one to cure you, Elise?' and, 'What did you do with the girls last night, Elise?' These comments would be pathetically funny if he'd only said them once or twice, but it's like a morning routine for him. I just freeze up when he comes into the office, and I'm ultra-paranoid that he's getting other people to laugh along with him. I feel that I've become the butt of the office jokes, and because I'm low, I'm making mistakes in my work.[15]

Conditions of Service

Many employers do not give the same conditions of service and benefits to lesbians and gay men as they do to heterosexual employees, especially married employees. Many employees in same sex relationships are not given any rights to, for example, compassionate leave, bereavement leave and pension entitlement. The lack of such rights can be extremely distressing when a partner becomes ill or dies.

The following example from LAGER demonstrates not only an uncaring attitude towards an employee who was ill with an HIV related illness, but also the way in which the partners of gay men do not have the legal status to claim employee benefits which are given to married partners of the opposite sex.

Mike had worked for an airline company for nearly two years. In December 1993 he was signed off work because of HIV related illnesses. His partner, Steve, looked after him while he was ill. Mike's absence from work continued until his death in July 1994. Mike's wages were paid until February 1994 and, after this time, negotiations took place between Mike's lawyer and the airline. It took the airline until 28 July to make an informal offer of a redundancy settlement to Mike. Mike was therefore without pay for five months whilst the airline was making its decision and Mike died before the settlement was secured.

Shortly after Mike's death, Steve tried to secure the redundancy payment for Mike's estate. The airline, however, withdrew the redundancy package by callously maintaining that Mike had frustrated his contract by dying!

At the time, there was nothing Steve could do legally to challenge their decision.[16]

Lesbians and Gay Men and Employment law

At the time of writing there is no specific protection for lesbians and gay men in employment law. In the past, people have been sacked, demoted, refused employment or promotion simply on the grounds that they are lesbian or gay. Although it is possible for a lesbian or a gay man to claim unfair dismissal at an industrial tribunal, there are past cases where tribunals have upheld decisions by employers to dismiss employees simply because of their sexuality.

The Two Year Rule

Because there is no specific protection for lesbians and gay men under employment law, lesbians and gay men must have worked for two years continuously with the same employer to qualify to take a case of unfair dismissal.

Sex Discrimination and Europe

In some circumstances, lesbians and gay men can claim under the Sex Discrimination Act (SDA) where there is no qualifying period of employment needed to take a case. However, the circumstances under which lesbians and gay men can claim sex discrimination are, at the time of writing, quite specific. The results of European rulings and further test cases will establish the extent to which discrimination on the grounds of sexuality can be challenged under the SDA.

It is also useful to note that, in 1991, the European Commission adopted a recommendation on the protection of the dignity of women and men at work, and a code of practice on measures to combat sexual harassment. The code specifically identifies lesbians and gay men among the groups particularly vulnerable to harassment. It states that it would be 'impossible to regard such harassment as appropriate workplace behaviour'. Although the recommendation is not legally binding, it is expected that tribunals would use it as an aid to interpreting the law where appropriate.

Harassment as a Criminal Offence

The Criminal Justice and Public Order Act 1994 introduced a new offence of intentional harassment on the grounds of race, sex, sexuality, age and disability. The Act includes harassment in the workplace. Employees who are harassed by work colleagues or by their employer are now in a position to report the matter to the police.

The Criminal Justice Act is the first piece of legislation in Britain to specifically include lesbians and gay men as one of the groups that should be given protection. It should be pointed out, however, that the practicalities of an employee calling the police and proving that they have been harassed are quite onerous.

Tribunal Attitudes

Despite the lack of specific protection for lesbians and gay men, there are some cases where tribunals have ruled in their favour. For example, a black gay man represented by LAGER won compensation at an industrial tribunal for constructive dismissal. LAGER reports:

> A black gay man employed by a travel company was frequently called abusive names by his manager such as 'Knobhead', 'Dickhead' and 'Cunt'. Every day he experienced comments about his genitalia. The employee said: 'The abuse ... lasted for over two years, despite liking the work I could no longer put up with my manager's insults, I was getting very embarrassed, very stressed and ill – I resigned.'
>
> The manager told the tribunal that he did not accept that the employee was upset by his comments and thought that he got on well with him. Medical evidence was given to the tribunal that the gay worker saw his doctor after and before he resigned. The doctor reported that the worker was in a severely anxious state as a result of his treatment at work.
>
> The tribunal decided that the manager had breached his duty of trust and confidence to the worker and that the claim for constructive dismissal therefore succeeded.[17]

What is Homophobia?

Homophobia is sometimes obvious, but it often manifests itself in very subtle ways. In the voluntary sector and 'caring professions' there is often a liberal tradition which prohibits blatant displays of homophobia, but its more subtle expressions often continue. In many other workplaces, homophobia is ingrained – from senior management to the staff canteen. See if any of the following sound familiar in your organisation.

- Assuming that everyone you meet is heterosexual, until you find out otherwise.

- Feeling that homosexuality and discussions about homophobia are unnecessary in workplace settings.

- Looking at lesbians, gay men and bisexuals and automatically thinking about their sexuality rather than seeing them as a whole, complex person.

- Thinking you can 'spot one'.

- Believing a lesbian is just a woman who could not find a man, or that a gay man must have been raped or sexually abused as a child.

- Thinking that if a lesbian or gay man touches you, she or he is making sexual advances.

- Wondering which one is 'the man' in a lesbian couple, or which one is 'the woman' in a gay male couple.

- Changing your seat in a meeting because you believe the person next to you is lesbian, gay or bisexual.

- Characterising lesbians as 'men-haters' or gay men as 'women-haters'.

- Feeling repulsed or uncomfortable seeing public displays of affection between lesbians or gay men but accepting the same displays of affection between heterosexuals as being nice or 'sweet'.

- Kissing an old friend, but hesitating to shake hands with a lesbian or a gay man.

- Using the terms 'lesbian' or 'gay' as accusations or insults.

- Not asking about the partner of a lesbian or a gay man even though you regularly ask 'How is your husband/wife/girlfriend/boyfriend?' when you run into a heterosexual friend.

- Avoiding mentioning to friends that you are friendly with a lesbian or a gay man in case they think you are lesbian, gay or bisexual.

- Failing to be supportive when a lesbian, a gay man or a bisexual friend is sad or upset about a quarrel, break-up or the death of a partner.

- Making sure everyone knows *you* are heterosexual whenever lesbian and gay issues are mentioned.

- Worrying about the effect a lesbian, gay or bisexual co-worker, volunteer, or client might have on your agency or business.

- Expecting a lesbian or a gay man to change her or his behaviour or mode of dress to work or socialise with you.

- Not confronting a homophobic remark because you are afraid of being labelled lesbian or gay.

- Feeling that lesbians and gay men are too outspoken about their rights.

By its very definition homophobia hurts everyone. Not only does it generate violence and discrimination against lesbians, gay men and bisexuals, it robs society of creative talents and contributions. For many people the fear of being labelled homosexual limits their behaviour and even career choices. Witness, for example, the widespread belief that all male hair stylists, nurses, decorators, artists and designers are gay. Or equally the belief that any woman who works in a job traditionally defined as 'men's work' – construction work, bus and train driving, engineering – must be a lesbian.

Taking into account the preceding details, a different, non-medical picture of HIV begins to emerge: HIV has been difficult to deal with not merely because of the science involved but because HIV appeared, grew and was nurtured in the cultural context of multiple discrimination, which further fed 'AIDSphobia'', which in turn further fed other forms of discrimination. Because of this, it is impossible to consider a rational approach to HIV without also confronting the realities that helped to make HIV so ominous, frightening and venomous.

HIV Diversity and the Workplace

What does all this mean for the workplace? A few essential points deserve to be made.

1. Discrimination is still with us; in fact it contaminates just about every aspect of modern life. It can rob organisations of the talents and contributions of lesbians and gay men, black people, people from ethnic minorities, women, disabled people and others.

2. HIV has brought the issue of homophobia to the forefront and addressing HIV means, by implication, addressing homophobia.

3. HIV and discrimination present a challenge to organisations: we can embrace diversity that forms the essence of modern society or we can run from it. It requires some courage, for example, for businesses to condemn homophobia and to openly welcome lesbian and gay staff and clients – especially if the surrounding community seems hostile to the idea. The alternative, however, is the continued condemnation of people for no other reason than who they love, their identity, skin colour or sex and losing out on the lessons that HIV really has to teach us.

4. Silence on the issue is complicity with discrimination. Organisations need to state openly what they believe so that all staff and clients are aware of, and working towards, the realisation of organisational values. The implication is clear: organisations will want to examine all areas of operations and evaluate whether they tend to promote or oppose the continuation of discrimination and thereafter put into place measures that will challenge and

condemn discrimination whenever and however it emerges.

Policy Recommendations

There are at several main policy implications that derive from the previous material.

1. It is evident that organisations need to ensure that their policies and procedures are designed to actively oppose HIV discrimination in the workplace. The rest of this book shows how such policies and procedures can be achieved.

2. Organisations will want to examine existing company policies that relate to equal opportunity in employment and services. Are they sufficiently inclusive? Do policies on race, sex and disability give detail about how discrimination is to be tackled? Are lesbians, gay men and bisexuals included in the organisation's equal opportunity statement? Do terms and conditions of service give equal benefits to same sex partners? Does the policy give staff and clients from diverse communities the right to equal and respectful treatment, care and services? If not, the equal opportunities policy statement should be revised so that it embraces such diversity.

3. Organisations will want to review their staff and, if appropriate, volunteer make-up, to assess the degree to which it adequately represents the demographic composition of the communities and client base it serves. If the organisation determines that the staff/volunteer make-up is too homogeneous, it should make special efforts to recruit and retain members of under-represented groups at all levels within the organisation.

4. Organisations will want to commit to the ongoing development of staff competence in relation to diversity issues. Such commitment should be integrated into policy and

planning to ensure that training and staff education are not prey to whoever is 'in charge' at any one moment. Some organisations may decide that training and education are too expensive because of the size and resources of the company. There are other options which can be explored. For example, some organisations have enjoyed considerable success in arranging 'training trades' with other organisations – this is where company A provides training for company B in A's area of expertise, and vice versa.

5. Organisations that are fully committed to opposing HIV related discrimination may also want to make a public statement about their anti-discrimination stance. There are two examples of the way that this can be achieved in relation to HIV. First, to adopt the statement of principles devised by the National AIDS Trust. The statement of principles is reproduced in Appendix 1 with information about how it can be adopted. Second, to sign the UK Declaration of the Rights of People with HIV and AIDS. The Declaration is reproduced in Appendix 2 along with information about how to support it.

7 Shaping Policy for Organisations

Introduction

Does the previous outline of HIV related topics relate to private companies, the public sector, the voluntary sector and trade unions? The answer is, mainly, yes. The essential substance of earlier chapters will be relevant to nearly every kind of organisation from the very small to the very large. Most organisations, however, will not need to concern themselves with those policy topics that seem to be related to the welfare of clients and residents, unless there is an application to employees. In other words, most corporate policy on HIV/AIDS will probably be simpler and less detailed than the HIV/AIDS policy one might find in, for example, a residential home for adults with mental health problems.

There are both positive and negative aspects to that fact. On the one hand, organisations will probably find that the actual development of HIV/AIDS policy will not require a great deal of effort. On the other hand (and unfortunately), too many organisations have responded to the challenge of AIDS by adopting policy that is too limited in scope, and therefore need to expand their thinking about the importance of truly comprehensive HIV policy.

Auditing HIV

This chapter provides a comprehensive range of information, techniques and instruments which can be used to assess where the organisation is now and what needs to be done in relation to HIV. In this sense the chapter provides all the tools necessary to conduct an HIV audit. The chapter is divided into four sections which contain the following:

Section One identifies the main areas which arise from the policy topics discussed in the previous chapters. A summary is given of the action organisations will need to take on these areas. A business checklist follows for readers to assess which policy areas are or are not being addressed in their organisation.

Section Two presents a range of pitfalls which need to be avoided if successful development and implementation of HIV policies are to be achieved. A questionnaire follows which can be used to give a more detailed assessment about areas which are or are not already being addressed in an organisation.

Section Three identifies six typical stages of development that an organisation may go through in its response to HIV/ AIDS. Identifying the stage that your organisation is currently at can be useful to determine the strategy and action needed to move on to further stages.

Section Four provides survey instruments which can used to conduct an HIV audit in any organisation. The questionnaires may also be useful as training resources. The survey instruments can be used to assess what stage (as identified in Section Three) the organisation is in; the knowledge and attitudes of staff (and, if appropriate, clients) in relation to HIV and beliefs and attitudes to homosexuality and bisexuality.

Section One: Policy Topics for Organisations

Information and Training

An organisation's management will find that it is in its best interest to provide all employees with sensitive, accurate, and effective education about HIV and AIDS. Not only can such education help to prevent potential disruption in the workplace, it can help to ensure that the workforce remains healthy

– which, in the long run, saves money. There are many sources of information and training available to organisations, and the cost of providing such information should be weighed against the benefits of preventing employee HIV infection and workplace crisis.

Employment Protection: Discrimination

Organisations will need to enact unambiguous policy prohibiting discrimination against any job applicant, employee, customer or contractee simply on the basis of that person's HIV status. In addition, management will need to examine corporate health and benefits packages to make sure that they treat HIV infection and AIDS in the same manner as any other chronic or potentially life-threatening illness, such as cancer or heart disease. Employees need to know that discrimination against or mistreatment of any other employee, because of perceived or real HIV antibody status, will not be tolerated. And employees living with HIV need to know that they can freely discuss matters related to health, performance, benefits or any other issues with appropriate personnel without fear of any form of reprisal.

Long-term and Intermittent Illnesses

Companies will want to ensure that they comply fully with the requirements of the Disability Discrimination Act, and to acknowledge that people with HIV related illnesses or disabilities are covered within the Act. Organisations that are committed to action on HIV will also recognise that being able to continue employment may be crucial for the well-being and self-esteem of a person who has a health problem related to their antibody status.

Confidentiality

Medical information about employees, including HIV antibody status, is legally protected, except in very rare cases. Organisations will need to formulate policy that safeguards the privacy of employees' medical information, in addition to shielding individuals from the sometimes harmful employee-to-employee gossip and rumour that can damage the smooth functioning of workplaces. Individuals with HIV related concerns should be encouraged to consult a designated, appropriate and named member of staff: any designated staff should have full training about HIV related matters and should always be able to give reassurance that unnecessary disclosure to others will not occur.

HIV Antibody Testing

It is difficult to imagine any circumstances in which routine testing of employees would be warranted, and as pointed out in an earlier chapter, such an action would be highly vulnerable to legal challenge. Organisations should take a firm position against mandatory testing of job applicants or employees, while at the same time providing all employees with accurate information about HIV antibody testing.

Universal Precautions

Infection control strategies in organisations will vary widely depending on the nature of the business. An organisation in the catering industry, for example, will no doubt have more stringent rules than a travel agency. The Health and Safety Executive can be consulted for assistance in developing business specific infection control policy. In many cases, specific policy has already been written, and can be adopted or adapted for use within a particular organisation.

Diversity/Equal Opportunities

And finally, organisations should recognise that part of the challenge of HIV is accepting, even embracing, the diversity of individuals in the workplace. We have already seen that HIV, at least to date, has had a disproportionate effect on gay men, black people and other minority groups that, even before HIV, suffered discrimination in communities and workplaces. The loss of talent and energy resulting from that discrimination has been enormous.

Organisations should view HIV as an opportunity to review their recruitment, hiring, retention and layoff practices to make sure that they respect and encourage the kind of diverse workforce that most experts are predicting as the reality of the future. Are lesbians and gay men protected by the corporate anti-discrimination policy? What about benefits for domestic partners? Do daily life and corporate culture in the workplace honour diversity?

Business Policy Checklist

Employment Protection: Discrimination

- ❑ Does policy prohibit discrimination against job applicants, employees, customers and contractors based on real or perceived HIV antibody status?

- ❑ Does policy guarantee fair access to company healthcare packages and benefits for people with HIV related illness?

Long-term and Intermittent Illnesses

- ❑ Are there any policies which deal with long-term and intermittent illnesses? Many companies have no policy on this area at all.

Confidentiality

- ❑ Does policy protect, according to law, the confidentiality of an employee's HIV status?

HIV Antibody Testing

- ❑ Does policy prohibit mandatory HIV antibody testing of employees or job applicants?

Infection Control/Universal Precautions

❑ Does policy spell out procedures for infection control in the workplace?

Employee Education/Training

❑ Does policy provide for effective education of all employees about HIV and AIDS?

Diversity

❑ Does policy provide protection against discrimination for lesbians, gay men and other groups?

❑ Does policy articulate methods for nurturing a corporate culture that embraces workplace diversity?

Section Two: Potential Traps and Pitfalls

In the process of developing and implementing comprehensive workplace HIV policy, organisations should guard against a number of common policy or strategic pitfalls. While certain obstacles to good HIV policy are also found in welfare or community orientated organisations, they are perhaps more likely to be seen in business settings. There are a number of reasons:

1. Workplaces, traditionally, are not forums for discussion about certain difficult, even intimate, matters such as sex, drugs and infectious disease.

2. The topic of HIV always, at some level, forces a certain set of values to the surface – about lesbians and gay men, about sexuality and moral belief, about trust and safety.

3. Addressing HIV and AIDS inevitably means facing the realities of sickness and death, and such personal loss is a very uncomfortable subject to confront.

4. And finally, discussion about HIV and AIDS, when conducted with people in their thirties and older, often brings up a host of fears and concerns about the safety, security – and sexuality – of our children, especially those who may be young adults and sexually active.

Pitfall 1:
Failing to Involve Representatives from All Levels of the Organisation in Policy Planning and Implementation – Line Workers and Top Management

If HIV policy planning does not include the perspectives of both the workers affected by policy and the managers who have the power to implement policy, the process will be marked by frustration and confusion, and the result will be only partially successful. The policy planning team should reflect the diversity of the organisation, while at the same time having enough vested authority to investigate problems, craft solutions and shepherd proposals through the corporate decision-making process with some reasonable chance of successful action.

Pitfall 2:
Allowing HIV Policy Making to be Cast as a 'Labour v. *Management' Debate*

An example from America helps to illustrate this point. A large organisation that had meat-packing operations as part of its business developed HIV policy addressing worksite infection control. This enterprise was also characterised by lukewarm relations between labour and management, and unfortunately management did not adequately consult with union representatives in the articulation and promulgation of HIV policy. Workers reacted to the policy announcement by asserting that 'management is not telling the whole truth' about AIDS in the workplace, and the policy initiative got muddled in all ensuing debates. In fact, the union ended up taking the issue to court (where their case was dismissed), and the labour/management polarisation was only heightened.

Workers and unions have historically believed that business has not and does not place a high enough value on occupational safety – and the contention is not without merit. Add to that the sometimes irrational fears that people still have about casual contact and HIV transmission, and it is not surprising that labour may sometimes reply, when told by management that 'there is no need to worry about HIV transmission in the workplace', with expressions of disbelief. Union representatives should always be involved in HIV policy planning.

Pitfall 3:
Failing to Allocate the Financial and Personnel Resources Required to Develop and Implement HIV Policy

Developing and implementing HIV policy in the workplace will require time and, ultimately, money. Freeing staff time for participation in the planning process, acquisition of materials, providing for employee education – all these carry a price tag.

It should be noted that the cost of HIV policy development and implementation is rarely excessive, that it is well within the capabilities of almost any concern, and that it always has to be measured against the costs of not doing anything. From the outset, management should commit the financial resources necessary to carry out policy planning and action.

Pitfall 4:
Adopting Policy Without Offering Employee Education about HIV; Offering Employee Education Without Good Policy to Back It Up

Some organisations have provided employees with good information about HIV but have failed to support that education with policy. Informing workers that 'there is no reason to treat people with HIV differently' in the workplace, but neglecting to underpin that information with anti-discrimination policy, will not help to eliminate discrimination in the long run. Similarly, if HIV discrimination is prohibited without educating employees about why it is prohibited, then anti-discrimination efforts will be undermined. HIV policy and employee education go hand in hand.

Pitfall 5:
Failing to Take into Account the Needs of Certain Operations, or Regional Differences Between Operations

Organisations with multiple sites and operations cannot expect that a single approach or even a single statement of policy on specific HIV topics, such as infection control, will work at every site, or for each operation. There are regional variations in style that must be taken into account when providing employee education; for example, the firm's lawyer from headquarters in London may not be the best person to give training to shop floor workers in Glasgow.

Policy makers in companies operating throughout Europe or internationally will also have to be aware of any legal variations between countries that may need to be taken into consideration.

Pitfall 6:
Approaching HIV in the Workplace as a 'One-Off' Issue, Rather than an Ongoing Concern Requiring Continual Monitoring

A number of organisations developed policies on HIV in the mid to late 1980s. Unfortunately some of these organisations (although by no means all) have not updated policies since that time. As a consequence, the policies will be factually out of date and may also use words and terms which are no longer appropriate.

In all matters related to HIV, the shifting landscape of law, healthcare management and research needs continual monitoring. Company policy makers need not only to survey current events in the world of HIV/AIDS, but to translate, when necessary, those events into revised company policy. The task is ongoing.

In addition, if an organisation provides employee education about HIV, that education should be a regular task as well. Not only are regular updates for all employees appropriate, but consideration should be given to employee turnover and ways in which the organisation can bring new workers up to speed on policy and the essential facts about HIV/AIDS.

Pitfall *7:* *Failing to Build Partnerships with Local and National HIV Organisations*

In almost every medium and large city in Europe, the United States and Canada there are local and national voluntary organisations providing HIV/AIDS education, training and information. HIV voluntary sector organisations have been in existence for years and they have been at the 'front-line' in the fight against HIV and AIDS. In so doing, they have accumulated enormous knowledge and expertise. Organisations that fail to tap into the available resources are neglecting a truly critical resource. HIV specific organisations are generally excellent resources to consult about the welfare and counselling services available to people affected by HIV. Some HIV organisations provide services directly aimed at employers and organisations who are trying to develop workplace initiatives in relation to HIV (see Appendix 1).

What keeps many businesses from forming partnerships with these voluntary organisations? It is certainly possible that some managers or policy makers are just not familiar with what is available. More likely, it is that many organisations simply aren't accustomed to building such 'private/voluntary sector' partnerships, or even considering them. Then, too, a certain degree of homophobia may be involved: many HIV service/education agencies have their roots in the gay community, and although they have become more diverse (as the epidemic began affecting many different populations), some people think of such agencies as 'gay identified' and want to keep a certain distance. None of these reasons, whether real or perceived, can justify any reservations about contacting groups who really know this epidemic, with all its intricacies.

Pitfall 8:
Approaching HIV Policy and Employee Education from a Purely 'Scientific', Detached Position

Some early education about HIV stuck to the 'scientific angle', attempting to carefully usher audiences through complex mazes of the science of HIV infection. While understanding that the facts are important, HIV educators soon learned that facts alone are not enough. Education and policy have to address the range of emotional responses that attend this condition, and help individuals to sort through personal feelings, values and beliefs to arrive at understanding, awareness and compassion.

Some organisations have recruited company medical personnel to deliver a 'science of HIV' lecture to employees. As long as the information is comprehensible to the audience, that is fine. But it is just as important to hear from people affected by HIV, or people with HIV related illnesses, about how infection or illness has affected their lives, and what support they need. It is equally important to allow dialogue, to engage people, to permit the free and open expression of feelings. Education that does not include such elements will only have limited effectiveness in the long run.

Pitfall 9:
'Sanitising' Employee Education about HIV and AIDS

One large organisation developed a comprehensive HIV policy and scheduled HIV education for all its employees. As part of the education session, a videotape about HIV and AIDS was shown. The video included interviews with a number of different people with HIV and AIDS, including openly gay men and a former heroin user, and presented those interviewees in a positive, supportive light.

Some employees objected: 'It's too gay'; 'It endorses homosexuality'; 'It doesn't condemn drug use strongly enough.' In reality, only a few people complained, but their voices were loud enough to cause management some concern.

Unfortunately in this case, management stopped using the video, and substituted one that was much more 'sanitary' in the eyes of the objectors. By doing so management chose to avoid some of the more controversial aspects of HIV and AIDS – and avoiding uncomfortable topics is part of what fuelled this epidemic in the first place.

HIV is about everybody: gay men, white suburban married couples, drug addicts, babies, prisoners, people with haemophilia, sex workers, managing directors. Preventing HIV infection, and providing good care for people with HIV disease, demands that we squarely face all the issues, not just those that are comfortable and 'safe'.

Pitfall 10:
Allowing HIV Policy and Employee Education to be Framed as an 'Us v. *Them' Dilemma*

Some individuals and groups of people have been cast as 'the bad guys' in this epidemic. One hears, for example, about bisexual men being 'responsible for bringing HIV into the heterosexual bedroom', and, unfortunately, some people still blame gay men for 'starting' this epidemic.

Any education or policy that perpetuates the belief that it is all 'us' (heterosexual, white, married, sober) versus 'them' (gay, bisexual, black people, drug users) ignores the fundamental reality: in this epidemic, 'Them' is 'Us'. Fostering hatred or animosity toward individuals or groups of people simply will not help in the long run and, in fact, may lead people to maintain mistaken, and potentially dangerous, attitudes (for example, 'Since I'm not gay or a drug user, I'm safe').

Assessing Workplace Readiness

Most business leaders are acutely aware that HIV is a significant workplace issue. Not only are many managers concerned with the safety, health and well-being of employees, they are also aware that situations involving HIV in the workplace, if badly handled, can prove disruptive and damage a company's ability to do business. Addressing HIV forthrightly is not only the right thing to do in terms of human impact, it is good business.

A large number of organisations will be affected by HIV in the coming years, and if they have not already, they will need to develop effective policy and educational responses. But how to start?

The following checklist[1] can help. It will allow a business to gain a sense of 'where we are', and, by implication, 'where we need to go'. It can be employed by individuals within a company who are attempting to start the process, or by teams that have a formal brief to work out what should be done in relation to HIV.

The questionnaire should be used in the following manner:

- Complete the questionnaire individually. If more than one person is completing it (for example, a policy team), average the responses.

- The survey's statements revolve around four basic topics related to HIV workplace readiness: 'Adjusting to Long-Term or Intermittent Illness', 'Discrimination', 'Confidentiality' and 'Health Maintenance'.

- Using the five-point response scale, circle the number corresponding to the response that best reflects your workplace's efforts to date. Respond to the statements from the perspective of your professional position.

- Identify what you think the 'next step' should be to improve your workplace's handling of each area of concern.

Questionnaire: Assessing Workplace Readiness

One: Adjusting to Long-term or Intermittent Illness

1 No workplace response

2 Inadequate workplace response

3 Adequate workplace response

4 Good workplace response

5 Exceptional workplace response

Circle one number:

A. Workplace education about HIV describes HIV related illness in the same context as other chronic long-term or intermittent illnesses.

1 2 3 4 5

B. Workplace policies anticipate the potential long-term productivity of HIV positive employees.

1 2 3 4 5

C. Terms and conditions relating to sickness are responsive to the chronic and cyclic nature of HIV related illnesses.

1 2 3 4 5

D. Managers are trained to provide reasonable adaptations for employees with HIV related illness.

1 2 3 4 5

E. Managers are trained to provide referrals to services that can help HIV positive employees.

1 2 3 4 5

F. Employees can use bereavement leave to cope with the loss of an unrelated partner, close friend or member of their work group.

1 2 3 4 5

Next steps:

Considering your responses to these statements, does your workplace need to improve its capacity to respond to HIV related illness as a chronic condition? What one or two activities should be considered priorities for next steps?

Two: Discrimination

1 No workplace response

2 Inadequate workplace response

3 Adequate workplace response

4 Good workplace response

5 Exceptional workplace response

Circle one number:

A. Policies prohibiting discrimination due to an employee's real or perceived HIV status are clear and unambiguous.

1 2 3 4 5

B. Education and training about discrimination are provided for all employees.

1 2 3 4 5

C. Discrimination due to real or perceived HIV status or sexuality is addressed as a part of HIV education or other education and training dealing with discrimination issues.

1 2 3 4 5

D. It has been clearly stated that employees with HIV illness will be afforded the same consideration as employees with other long-term or intermittent illnesses.

1 2 3 4 5

E. Managers have been trained to understand the workplace application of laws protecting employees with disabilities.

1 2 3 4 5

F. Policies prohibiting discrimination on the grounds of being lesbian or gay are clear and unambiguous.

1 2 3 4 5

Next steps:

Considering your responses to these statements, does your workplace need to improve its capacity to respond to HIV discrimination? What one or two activities should be considered priorities for next steps?

Three: Confidentiality

1 No workplace response

2 Inadequate workplace response

3 Adequate workplace response

4 Good workplace response

5 Exceptional workplace response

Circle one number:

A. Procedures for handling confidential information are clearly defined.

1 2 3 4 5

B. Compliance with procedures for managing confidential medical and personal information is regularly monitored.

1 2 3 4 5

C. Employees who handle confidential medical and personal information have participated in HIV related education and training.

1 2 3 4 5

D. Steps have been taken to inform and reassure all employees that medical and personal information is handled confidentially.

1 2 3 4 5

E. Managers have been trained to understand and implement 'need to know' standards regarding confidential medical and personal information.

1 2 3 4 5

Next steps:

Considering your responses to these statements, does your workplace need to improve its capacity to respond to HIV confidentiality? What one or two activities should be considered priorities for next steps?

Four: Health Maintenance

1 No workplace response

2 Inadequate workplace response

3 Adequate workplace response

4 Good workplace response

5 Exceptional workplace response

Circle one number:

A. Good practice in regard to health and safety is encouraged for all employees.

1 2 3 4 5

B. Company pension schemes do not require information about an employee's HIV status.

1 2 3 4 5

C. Company pension schemes give equal benefits to same sex partners.

1 2 3 4 5

D. Company health insurance treats all long-term and intermittent illnesses equally.

1 2 3 4 5

E. Comprehensive workplace education about HIV is regularly offered to all employees.

1 2 3 4 5

Next steps:

Considering your responses to these statements, does your workplace need to improve its capacity to respond to HIV and health maintenance? What one or two activities should be considered priorities for next steps?

Section Three: Organisational Stages

Before an organisation can change – that is, develop appropriate rules and regulations and nurture the skills required to implement those policies – it must have a clear understanding of:

1. Where the organisation is – an analysis of the current situation;

2. Where the organisation wants to be – a sense of goals and vision; and

3. A plan for what the organisation will do – a strategy for getting there.

A central part of the organisation's analysis of itself, in relation to being prepared for HIV/AIDS, will involve a determination of its current stage. Most organisations go through a series of clear, definable stages in their response to HIV/AIDS. An understanding of those stages can aid the professional in analysing the organisation's current condition and charting desirable futures. The work in this section is drawn from experience with hundreds of organisations – no doubt the reader will be able to recognise, somewhere in the stages, her or his organisation. There are six stages in all:

- Consciousness;
- Concern;
- Crisis;
- Containment;
- Collaboration;
- Commitment.

Organisations tend to move in a more or less linear fashion through the stages, starting at the first stage and 'arriving', at some point in the future, at the sixth. Each stage has distinct features, and most organisations tend to be 'at' one stage at a time, but there is some fluidity between the boundaries. In the following discussion, each stage is outlined in turn, and described in terms of:

1. Its general features;
2. The feelings, talk, and action that typify that stage; and
3. The precipitating events that often move the organisation from the previous stage to the current one.

Stage One: *Consciousness*

GENERAL FEATURES

- Rudimentary awareness of a reality called HIV as something 'out there', in some place or setting other than the organisation.
- People in the organisation are also likely to believe that many of the faces of HIV (gay men, intravenous drug users, etc.) live elsewhere, outside the organisational reality. This belief is rarely checked for accuracy; it is simply an unquestioned assumption, resting on the premise that 'if I don't know about it, it doesn't exist'. Comments are made such as:

" We've never had any gays working here, as far as I know. I think I'd know something like that.

" Yes, I've heard about HIV, but I don't think about it very much.

FEELINGS, TALK, ACTION

- Very little discussion of HIV or HIV related issues in the organisation – no compelling reason for such discussions. When mentioned at all, it is generally in the same tones people adopt for talking about hunger in Africa: distant, regrettable, but easily ignored.

- The facts about HIV, and the implications of those facts for organisational life, are not yet a regular part of the organisation's agenda.

- It is doubtful that there is any action at all at this stage. There is nothing yet to act towards or against. HIV is merely a part of consciousness, something of which people are aware, but nothing more.

MOVEMENT FROM PREVIOUS STAGE: PRECIPITATING EVENT(S)

If there were a previous stage, it would have to be 'never heard of HIV or AIDS at all'. Now, in the 1990s, it is difficult to imagine a business or social service professional who has not heard at least something. In some ways, that is an advantage over the early 1980s: almost everyone now knows that HIV and AIDS exist.

Stage Two: *Concern*

GENERAL FEATURES

- A generalised awareness that 'AIDS is possible here'. It is no longer a mere abstraction, but a real potential. In this stage, it has not happened yet, but members of the organisation are aware that it could.

FEELINGS, TALK, ACTION

- Discrete and recognisable feelings about HIV or AIDS and HIV related issues start to surface. People may become aware of their fear.

- They may feel angry at gay men, at the government, at society as a whole for making them have to think about HIV and how it affects them.

" It's that sexual revolution thing. If it weren't for everybody jumping into bed all the time we wouldn't have this. I've been moral, but others ...

- At this stage sometimes profound and persistent feelings of guilt and shame can emerge (or re-emerge) especially about past sexual behaviour or past use of intravenous drugs. Those feelings may appear as fears about possible acquisition of HIV, but the underlying issue is unresolved guilt.

" Ten years ago I had a brief affair. It was nothing, meant nothing, so I never told my husband, and he never found out about it. Now I'm sure I've got AIDS because of it.

- The range of feelings that can begin to arise will be unique to different members of the organisation. Some may feel hopeless, others helpless. Some may feel sad at the toll HIV is exacting, at the 'loss of collective innocence' and so on. Still others may feel relatively little or nothing.

- It is important to note that the general concern of this stage can have positive, as well as not-so-positive, roots: it may indicate for some, a sense of confusion and protectiveness; for others, a more compassionate concern that the reality of HIV is threatening all of us.

- People do begin talking more openly about HIV in the organisation, but the dialogues are directionless, diffuse expressions of feelings for which there is little resulting action.

" I keep thinking we should do something to get ready, in case it happens. I do not know what we'll do if it does.

- What little action there is in this stage is often poorly planned or carried out. Revised infection control procedures, for example, may be published, but they are unevenly implemented. Staff may be very careful with a client known to have a history of intravenous drug use, for example, and careless with clients with an unknown risk history. Client education is sometimes started, but because the overall organisational focus is unclear, the education is hit-or-miss, without an underlying philosophy or goals.

MOVEMENT FROM PREVIOUS STAGE: PRECIPITATING EVENT(S)

There are a number of events that are likely to precipitate movement from Consciousness to Concern. They include, but are certainly not limited to, the following:

- The organisation accepts a client who has a 'high risk' history (for example, someone who has used intravenous drugs in the recent past), but who is nevertheless HIV antibody negative.
- The local community becomes aware of its first (known) resident with HIV. Especially in smaller towns and cities, this can have a dramatic effect on other residents.
- The organisation may receive guidelines from the government or another agency. Even in the local absence of HIV infection, such guidelines can 'force the issue' of future potential.
- Staff may discover family members, even distant relatives, who have HIV.
- Staff may begin hearing of organisations similar to theirs, with roughly the same mission and goals, that 'now have people with AIDS' among their caseloads or on the staff.

The above examples all point to a common feature: something has happened to make the possibility of HIV become tangible.

Stage Three: *Crisis*

GENERAL FEATURES

- Crisis is the most distinct of all the stages; it is launched by a very specific occurrence: the known presence or impending presence of HIV in the 'organisational family'. It matters little whether the infected person is among staff or clients, whether she or he is symptomatic. What matters is that the Human Immunodeficiency Virus is inside the four walls of the organisation.

- Crisis does not necessarily connote visible disruption as much as a profound conflict of beliefs, norms, goals and values, all of which may play itself out on internal arenas. If everyone is acutely frightened and confused, even if they are not talking about it, it is still a kind of crisis and demands intervention and management.

- Few organisations will be immune from some crisis in relation to HIV/AIDS. Trying to circumvent or bury HIV related organisational crisis will prove fruitless; in fact, if anything, such a crisis provides an extraordinary opportunity for new growth and development.

FEELINGS, TALK, ACTION

- Feelings are high in Stage Three, and often entirely unpredictable. The feelings themselves are nothing new – they will be familiar from Stage Two – but the intensity has increased. At times they threaten to, or actually do, boil over, as when staff meetings are made chaotic with sharp expressions of anger or frustration. Usually, however, they are not quite so obvious; they come out in staff conversations, in supervisory meetings, or indirectly through behaviour. Some staff members may threaten to leave 'if we take on someone who has AIDS'.

- Some staff members may threaten to refuse service to an infected client or to work with an infected co-worker.

- Staff in charge of the recruitment of employees or the admission of clients may consider refusing someone who is known to be antibody positive. Of course, staff can always 'veil' reasons for refusing someone, citing a long list of other reasons.

- Some staff members may begin covertly or overtly lobbying for their 'rights', generally for 'a safe working environment'. Superficially this sounds reasonable, and is in fact a justified request from employees. Often though, when it comes to HIV, this may translate into a demand for an impossible guarantee that there will never be any danger of infection for employees, any time, under any conditions.

" I'm tired of hearing about the rights of those people. What about my rights! Can you prove there will never be a danger!

- Some staff may exhibit a tendency to overstate risk, and therefore grossly over-compensate in taking health and safety precautions.

- There may be a polarisation between staff and management or clients and staff, because people feel 'forced' into something they do not want, or feel that they are not being told everything they 'need' to know.

- There tend to be lots of hushed conversations where people feed off one another's anxieties and anger.

- The organisation may arrange 'emergency' meetings or training with the expectation that it can 'nip the problem in the bud' quickly and decisively.

" We're getting our first client with AIDS tomorrow afternoon. Can you come in and do a quick one-hour training for all the staff and clients tomorrow morning?

- A host of HIV related issues may come to the fore, with a previously unknown depth and ferocity. For example, latent homophobic feelings and attitudes, or judgemental responses to sex workers, intravenous drug users or other affected groups may surface.

- Or, in something of a contradiction to much of the above, the organisation may experience a thorough and strained silence. It might be that no one says anything, but the tension is entirely evident.

> " When our first HIV positive client came, no one said anything. You'd think people would have a lot to say, but they didn't. You could feel it, though; you could cut it with a knife.

The list of possible organisational responses in the midst of crisis is seemingly endless. Crisis, by its very nature, generates a myriad list of options and reactions. Often HIV related crises elicit 'negative' responses, but such is not always the case. An organisation might also respond in more positive, helpful ways.

- Some staff, if characterised by a great deal of maturity and cohesive trust, could collectively decide to confront fears as fears – nothing more and nothing less – rather than as unalterable truth.
- Planning may be sufficient to foresee many of the problems and dilemmas that would attend the actual presence of HIV, and already have in place contingencies that will mitigate the worst of negative responses.

MOVEMENT FROM PREVIOUS STAGE: PRECIPITATING EVENT(S)

There is, as already noted, only one event that produces Stage Three, 'Crisis': the actual presence, or impending entry, of HIV in the organisation.

***Stage Four**: Containment*

GENERAL FEATURES

In the face of competing demands and tangible conflict, organisations generally tend toward solutions that address the lowest common denominators. They deal with symptoms and shy away from underlying causes. In the case of HIV, that process can be called containment: minimally adapting to the crisis in order to tame the worst of collective worries and fears. Because the most visible aspects of crisis have been addressed – but not the underlying dilemmas – the central feature of an organisation in Stage Four, 'containment' is continuing, unresolved conflict.

FEELINGS, TALK, ACTION

The feelings, talk and action of Stage Four all tend to betray the presence of unresolved conflict and lingering dilemmas.

- Managers may arrange ongoing HIV education for all staff and clients, but it emphasises the epidemiological or virological aspects of HIV infection, ignoring its social, sexual, political and ethical aspects.

- The organisation will have in place a number of HIV related policies, but they are inconsistently implemented and monitored.

- Staff enact different rules for other staff or clients who are known to be HIV positive from those for people whose antibody status is not known.

- Risk reduction education efforts may be targeted only toward clients, ignoring the sexual or drug-taking lives of staff.

- Attitudes about HIV are still death focused, rather than focused on life and maintaining life.

- Attitudes about lesbians and gay men, or members of other HIV affected communities are based on an uneasy tolerance.

" I know that Jack's gay, and he's okay. But I have to say I feel a little funny when he brings his lover to staff parties. I just never know what to say.

- Older organisational contradictions that are somehow related to AIDS and HIV begin to emerge. For example, staff working with people with mental health problems or developmental disabilities are sometimes uncomfortable with the idea that their clients may be sexually active, and may deny such activity takes place. It is not uncommon to hear the comment: 'Our clients don't have sex'.

- There are many old, unresolved dilemmas in the fields of caring and welfare, especially about sexuality and the nature of 'acceptable' sexual behaviour.

MOVEMENT FROM PREVIOUS STAGE: PRECIPITATING EVENT(S)

Movement from Stage Three to Stage Four occurs not so much because of discrete events as because of the desire to avoid some of the discomfort and anguish that the crisis stage can bring. There are, however, a number of factors that will predispose an organisation toward a 'containment' strategy in the face of HIV related crisis.

- The organisation has little or no history of dealing with some of the thornier HIV related issues, i.e. sexuality and homophobia.

- The organisation is typified by a crisis management style that elevates narrow, short-term interests over long-term, broad considerations.

- The organisation has done little or no advance training about HIV and HIV related issues.

- The organisation may be marked by a relative degree of mistrust among staff members; their work style might be characterised as more competitive than co-operative.

Unfortunately, many agencies reach Stage Four and stay there, without real change. Since legal obligations are satisfied, and the overt 'crisis' has been quelled, the organisation's task, on the surface, is done. Tired perhaps of dealing with crisis, afraid perhaps of doing some of the hard work that real change will require, everyone wants to get back to 'business as usual'. The underlying problems are still there, however, and the organisation that stays in Stage Four will miss out on the greater opportunities for growth that HIV/AIDS offers.

Stage Five: *Collaboration*

GENERAL FEATURES

Collaboration is characterised by an increasing dissatisfaction with the net results of 'containment', coupled with a growing ability to articulate underlying difficulties and devise the means for resolving those difficulties. In many ways, it is a transitional stage. Private disagreements and animosity are increasingly replaced with a more collaborative stance, a growing sense that everyone needs to be involved in the development of a long-term philosophy and strategy that will work. On its most basic level, people in Stage Five have begun to look beyond narrow personal fears and interests, and have begun to re-examine the organisation's goals and mission in the light of a now long-established, universally impacting disease.

FEELINGS, TALK, ACTION

As a distinctly transitional stage, collaboration is marked by feelings, talk and action that waver between progress and regression, between forward momentum and stagnation, between hope and resignation. What underlies the variations is a subtle change in perception.

- There is a growing awareness that homophobia, racism, sexism and other forms of oppression underlie the HIV issue.

" Every time I talk to clients about HIV, all the 'bender jokes' start coming out. I'm beginning to realise that we have to deal with that. It seems really difficult to talk about HIV without talking about some of that.

- Individuals come to recognise the personal issues that commonly surface when fighting HIV: fear of mortality, images of 'infection' and 'disease', struggles with the nature of intimacy (and so on). Such issues are increasingly identified and claimed as personal difficulties.

- Individuals come to see that with HIV, 'pulling on the threads unravels the whole fabric'. That is, they will move away from specific, unrelated observations and toward more holistic analyses.

- Members of the organisation catch glimpses of the opportunity that HIV presents, not just the threat.

" The more I talk to people with HIV the more I realise that I have a lot to learn about death, about dying, about living. This sounds weird, but I sometimes find myself grateful for that.

- Finally, people begin to imagine the unimaginable, to form organisational visions hitherto unarticulated: 'an organisation free of bias, nurturing everyone's individuality and uniqueness'; 'an agency that serves as a model in the fight against HIV'. Members of the organisation may not state the vision in precisely those terms, but the initial content will be there.

MOVEMENT FROM PREVIOUS STAGE: PRECIPITATING EVENT(S)

- The organisation may experience a change in key leadership that brings in someone strong, charismatic and visionary, someone with the necessary organisational skills to realise a vision. Experience informs us that almost every organisation that moves beyond Stage Four is headed by effective, sensitive, proactive management.

- The organisation may experience the death or hear of the infection of a client or staff person who is popular, well loved. When the client or staff person is not well known or liked, it is easier to distance oneself from the experience;

when strong attachments are present, it is much harder to 'contain' the feelings. It may appear callous to diminish the sickness or death of someone – anyone – but our experience certainly bears this out: if you do not know or like someone, their sickness or death will have considerably less impact.

- In larger organisations, with a number of clients or staff who are infected or ill, their persistent lobbying and self-advocacy stating, 'this is not good enough' may force the organisation out of containment.

- The organisation may be forced out of complacent containment by legal action that charges discrimination or substandard treatment for those living with HIV.

Stage Six: *Commitment*

GENERAL FEATURES

Stage Six is difficult to characterise, partly because there are few organisations to which one can point as models, and partly because this stage is not so neatly marked by definitive features. Commitment is, ultimately, a vision of the best an organisation can be in the fight against HIV/AIDS.

FEELINGS, TALK, ACTION

- Rather than mere acceptance, or even resignation to fate, the organisation actually welcomes people with HIV or AIDS as clients and as staff. The group does so first of all because the need exists, and it is within the mission of every private, public and voluntary organisation to serve the well being of its clients and staff; and secondly, the organisation consciously embraces the learning and growth that can come from diversity.

- The organisation is committed to developing the in-house expertise that will allow it to serve people with HIV or AIDS well. It will not 'shunt off' the above people to HIV service organisations every time they experience an HIV related need. Thus, for example, the organisation could develop and sponsor an in-house HIV positive support group if there is a sufficient number of staff or clients affected.

- Necessary procedures, such as infection control, are in place, and are followed calmly, without undue fear, by all.
- The organisation is committed to the ongoing education of all staff and clients, aimed not at 'filling your head with facts', but rather with the goal of helping each person to develop their innate ability to separate fact from fiction, and make appropriate decisions accordingly.
- The organisation recognises and affirms that when it comes to HIV, it is not a matter of 'us *vs.* them', it is only us – all staff, management, clients. That recognition is both personal and professional.
- The organisation is cognisant of the underlying realities of HIV (homophobia, racism, sexism, fear of sexuality and intimacy, and so on) and is committed to taking progressive steps that will eventually eradicate them from organisational life. Staff and clients will address personal issues, like fears about mortality, *as* personal issues.
- The organisation has a long-range plan addressing HIV and HIV related issues that encompasses service demands, special needs, resource management, education and all other areas.
- The organisation has come to recognise long-standing organisational contradictions preventing progress in the fight against HIV, and is taking active steps to resolve those contradictions.

MOVEMENT FROM PREVIOUS STAGE: PRECIPITATING EVENT(S)

No decisive event will move any organisation from Stage Five into Stage Six. It is a process. The fruits of Stage Six are likely to be achieved over time by hard work, strong leadership and committed staff. Without those elements, Stage Six will remain elusive, unattainable.

Where would you place your organisation on this continuum of stages? An accurate assessment of your organisation, in this regard, will be crucial to the process of policy development and, especially, implementation. Instruments designed to gauge organisational stage status follows in the next section.

Section Four: Survey Instruments

The following questionnaires will be useful for assessing, on a number of levels, your organisation's 'state of being' in relation to HIV/AIDS and its attendant issues. At the very least you are encouraged to use the first two; you can add the additional surveys as you feel they are appropriate or desirable. Of course, the more information you can gather about your organisation, the more effectively you can plan policy and procedures.

All the surveys should be administered anonymously, and if used, should be administered to all staff. Strict confidentiality should be assured for all participants and adhered to.

On subsequent pages you will find the following questionnaires:

1. 'HIV and the Organisation' is designed to determine, overall, the 'stage' your business or organisation is at. It takes only 5–10 minutes to complete. Scoring procedures follow the survey.

2. The 'HIV/AIDS Questionnaire' will tell you a lot about an individual's knowledge and attitudes about HIV/AIDS and HIV/AIDS related issues. The scoring procedure follows the questionnaire.

3. 'Beliefs and Attitudes about Bisexuality/Homosexuality'

will reveal aggregate attitudes about bisexuals, gay men and lesbians, and certain aspects concerning bisexuality and homosexuality. Research has indicated, over and over again, that there is a strong correlation between how people perceive bisexual/gay/lesbian people and how they perceive people with HIV/AIDS; if they are accepting of one group, it is very likely that they will be accepting of the other, and vice versa. At any rate, working with people with HIV/AIDS will force people, inevitably, to confront beliefs and values about bisexuality/homosexuality. Comments on interpreting the survey follow.

Much of the scoring is based on the assumption that some responses are more desirable than others, rather than absolutes of right or wrong. Desirable answers indicate, for the most part, the respondents' degree of comfort with a subject.

HIV and the Organisation

Please indicate which description seems to most accurately describe your organisation's current approach or stance towards HIV and AIDS. Tick only one.

- ❑ We've had people (staff or clients) here with HIV or AIDS, and have done some education and policy development in response. The education isn't very interesting; it's mostly medical. Generally staff have a lot of pity for people who have HIV or AIDS because it's so sad that they are going to die. Overall, the situation seems pretty much under control.

- ❑ Most people realise that we could see HIV in our organisation, but it hasn't happened yet, as far as I know. At first, it seemed far away, but now it seems as if it's getting closer and closer all the time. We probably should do more to get ready but it seems a little overwhelming. It has made me think about whether I'm at risk, or other people I know are at risk.

- ❑ There has been very little discussion about HIV/AIDS within my organisation. It doesn't seem terribly likely that we will ever get anyone with HIV here, so we've never done anything with education or policy. It's not that we don't care, it's just that it doesn't affect us.

- ❑ I think working with people with HIV has been a great learning experience for us, and, in a strange way, I'm grateful. I feel that I know a lot about HIV and I'm learning more all the time; it's been a personally developing experience. I know it has made us look at some of the ways 'we've always done things', and ask hard questions. More and more I value diversity: gays and straights, men and women, black and white people.

- ❑ We've worked with people with HIV, and have done quite a bit. More and more, however, it seems as if we're missing some of the bigger issues, like how people feel about sex or gay people. A lot of beliefs and values come up when we discuss HIV and they're not being talked about enough. I know that I've begun thinking about it differently, maybe we can learn something from all this.

- ❑ We've recently found out that someone here (staff or clients) has AIDS. It seems to have had quite an effect on people. I've noticed that some people have strong feelings about it, and there have been a few problems. I don't think we really have the situation under control yet.

HIV and the Organisation: Scoring

Each of the statements on the survey corresponds to the perspective one would be likely to have at each of the six stages. Notice that the order here is different from the survey.

- ❑ There has been very little discussion about HIV/AIDS within my organisation. It doesn't seem terribly likely that we will ever get anyone with HIV here, so we've never done anything with education or policy. It's not that we don't care, it's just that it doesn't affect us.

This corresponds to Stage One, Consciousness. Mark here for each respondent who ticked it. ____

- ❑ Most people realise that we could see HIV in our organisation, but it hasn't happened yet, as far as I know. At first, it seemed far away, but now it seems as if it's getting closer and closer all the time. We probably should do more to get ready but it seems a little overwhelming. It has made me think about whether I'm at risk, or other people I know are at risk.

This corresponds to Stage Two, Concern. Mark here for each respondent who ticked it. ____

- ❑ We've recently found out that someone here (staff or clients) has AIDS. It seems to have had quite an effect on people. I've noticed that some people have strong feelings about it, and there have been a few problems. I don't think we really have the situation under control yet.

This corresponds to Stage Three, Crisis. Mark here for each respondent who ticked it. ____

- ❑ We've had people (staff or clients) here with HIV or AIDS, and have done some education and policy development in response. The education isn't very interesting; it's mostly medical. Generally staff have a lot of pity for people who have HIV or AIDS because it's so sad that they're going to die. Overall, the situation seems pretty much under control.

This corresponds to Stage Four, Containment. Mark here for each respondent who ticked it. ____

- ❑ We've worked with people with HIV, and have done quite a bit. More and more, however, it seems as if we're missing some of the bigger issues, like how people feel about sex or gay people. A lot of beliefs and values come up when we discuss HIV and they're not being talked about enough. I know that I've begun thinking about it differently, maybe we can learn something from all this.

This corresponds to Stage Five, Collaboration. Mark here for each respondent who ticked it. ____

- ❑ I think working with people with HIV has been a great learning experience for us, and, in a strange way, I'm grateful. I feel that I know a lot about HIV and I'm learning more all the time; it's been a personally developing experience. I know it has made us look at some of the ways 'we've always done things', and ask hard questions. More and more I value diversity: gays and straights, men and women, black and white people.

This corresponds to Stage Six, Commitment. Mark here for each respondent who ticked it. ____

It is quite unlikely that everyone will answer the same way. You will notice, however, a general grouping around one or two stages. That will give you a fairly accurate picture of how people in the organisation see themselves, in relation to the stages.

HIV/AIDS Questionnaire

1. How much do you know about the Human Immunodeficiency Virus (HIV) and Acquired Immune Deficiency Syndrome (AIDS)? Tick one.

    ❑ A great deal
    ❑ A certain amount
    ❑ Very little
    ❑ Nothing

2. Identify the statement that best describes your feelings about HIV/AIDS. Tick one.

    ❑ I don't really need to know anything about HIV/AIDS.
    ❑ I need to learn about HIV/AIDS, but it really doesn't affect me or my family.
    ❑ I want to learn about HIV/AIDS. It may affect me or people I love.
    ❑ I want to learn about HIV/AIDS. It's affecting everybody.

3. What have been your sources of information about HIV/AIDS? Tick all that apply.

    ❑ Television or radio
    ❑ Newspapers or magazines
    ❑ Pamphlets or brochures
    ❑ Members of my family

- ❑ Friends or co-workers
- ❑ Teachers or lecturers
- ❑ Ministers or other spiritual leaders
- ❑ Doctors or other medical personnel
- ❑ Professional HIV/AIDS educators
- ❑ The Internet

4. How concerned are you about acquiring HIV at work? Tick one.

- ❑ I am very concerned
- ❑ I am moderately concerned
- ❑ I am a little concerned
- ❑ I am not at all concerned

5. How concerned are you about acquiring HIV because of your own sexual or drug-using behaviour? Tick one.

- ❑ Very concerned
- ❑ Moderately concerned
- ❑ A little concerned
- ❑ Not at all concerned

6. Do you know or have you ever known someone with HIV infection or AIDS? Tick one.

- ❑ Yes
- ❑ I believe so, but I'm not sure
- ❑ No

7. If 'yes' that person is/was (tick one):

- ❑ A sexual partner
- ❑ An intravenous-drug using partner
- ❑ A member of my immediate family
- ❑ Someone in my extended family
- ❑ A close friend
- ❑ A friendly acquaintance
- ❑ Just someone I knew of

For questions 8–27, circle the answer you believe to be correct or closest to the truth.

8. Currently, all blood donated for transfusions is screened for the HIV antibody.

   TRUE FALSE UNSURE

9. You can get HIV infection by drinking from the same glass as someone who has HIV.

   TRUE FALSE UNSURE

10. If you share intravenous drug injection equipment with another person you are at risk of HIV infection.

    TRUE FALSE UNSURE

11. You can get HIV from a mosquito bite.

    TRUE FALSE UNSURE

12. You can become infected with HIV by donating blood.

    TRUE FALSE UNSURE

13. A woman infected with HIV can pass the virus on to her unborn child.

    TRUE FALSE UNSURE

14. People sharing a flat with someone who is HIV infected are at high risk of acquiring the disease.

    TRUE FALSE UNSURE

15. A 'positive' blood test means that one is infected with HIV.

    TRUE FALSE UNSURE

16. Staff who are working closely with clients who are HIV infected are at greatly elevated risk of contracting the disease.

    TRUE FALSE UNSURE

17. There are clinics in most cities and large towns where an individual may go for a confidential or anonymous HIV antibody test.

    TRUE FALSE UNSURE

18. You can tell just by looking at someone whether or not they are HIV infected.

    TRUE FALSE UNSURE

19. Individuals can pass HIV to others without knowing it.

    TRUE FALSE UNSURE

20. HIV can be sexually transmitted from man to man, man to woman, woman to man and woman to woman.

    TRUE FALSE UNSURE

21. You can get HIV infection from French kissing.

    TRUE FALSE UNSURE

22. Use of condoms can significantly reduce the chance of infection, if used properly every time one has sexual intercourse.

    TRUE FALSE UNSURE

23. If one is not gay/bisexual or an intravenous drug user, one doesn't really need to worry about HIV or AIDS.

    TRUE FALSE UNSURE

24. AIDS is now curable.

TRUE FALSE UNSURE

25. Tears and sweat are HIV infectious.

TRUE FALSE UNSURE

26. Receiving blood donations is now safe from the chance of HIV infection.

TRUE FALSE UNSURE

27. One should be careful when choosing a doctor or dentist because they could have AIDS and transmit it to their patients.

TRUE FALSE UNSURE

For questions 28–50 circle the number that seems to correspond most accurately to your reaction to the statement.

Strongly disagree		*Not sure*		*Strongly agree*
1	2	3	4	5

28. Our organisation should find out about the health of the people it employs.

1 2 3 4 5

29. Our organisation should find out about the health of its clients.

1 2 3 4 5

30. I am entitled to know if a co-worker or client has HIV or AIDS.

1 2 3 4 5

Strongly disagree *Not sure* *Strongly agree*

1 2 3 4 5

31. I have the right to a transfer if a client or co-worker has HIV or AIDS.

1 2 3 4 5

32. People with HIV/AIDS should be allowed to live in a residential home.

1 2 3 4 5

33. Homosexuality should not be a cause for discrimination in any situation.

1 2 3 4 5

34. People with HIV/AIDS have the right to work in hospitals.

1 2 3 4 5

35. There are many people with HIV/AIDS who are spreading the virus on purpose.

1 2 3 4 5

36. People with HIV/AIDS should be permanently separated from the rest of society.

1 2 3 4 5

37. To some extent, people who contract HIV through sex or intravenous drug use deserve it.

1 2 3 4 5

38. People with HIV or AIDS should be barred from teaching.

1 2 3 4 5

Strongly disagree		*Not sure*		*Strongly agree*
1	2	3	4	5

39. I doubt that anyone I know will get HIV infected.

    1 2 3 4 5

40. People with HIV or AIDS have the right to anonymity.

    1 2 3 4 5

41. Homosexuality is not acceptable to me.

    1 2 3 4 5

42. People with HIV or AIDS should be prohibited from working with food in restaurants.

    1 2 3 4 5

43. It is extremely doubtful that any of our clients will get HIV or AIDS.

    1 2 3 4 5

44. Intravenous drug users do not care about anything but their 'fix'.

    1 2 3 4 5

45. A person with HIV who doesn't inform their sexual partner should be jailed.

    1 2 3 4 5

46. I have personally changed some of my behaviours because of HIV.

    1 2 3 4 5

Strongly disagree		*Not sure*		*Strongly agree*
1	2	3	4	5

47. Scientists who say that HIV can't be spread by casual contact don't really have all the facts they claim to have.

1 2 3 4 5

48. Doctors with HIV should always tell their patients of their infection.

1 2 3 4 5

49. There should be a law requiring testing for everyone; that way, we'll know for certain.

1 2 3 4 5

50. Homosexuality is a serious threat to our cherished values and institutions.

1 2 3 4 5

HIV/AIDS Questionnaire: Scoring

Write in number ticked in the box [ ].

1. How much do you know about the Human Immunodeficiency Virus (HIV) and Acquired Immune Deficiency Syndrome (AIDS)? Tick one.

❑ A great deal [ ]
❑ A certain amount [ ]
❑ Very little [ ]
❑ Nothing [ ]

2. Identify the statement that best describes your feelings about HIV/AIDS. Tick one.

   - ❑ I don't really need to know anything about HIV/AIDS. [ ]
   - ❑ I need to learn about HIV/AIDS, but it really doesn't affect me or my family. [ ]
   - ❑ I want to learn about HIV/AIDS. It may affect me or people I love. [ ]
   - ❑ I want to learn about HIV/AIDS. It's affecting everybody. [ ]

3. What have been your sources of information about HIV/AIDS? Tick all that apply.

   - ❑ Television or radio [ ]
   - ❑ Newspapers or magazines [ ]
   - ❑ Pamphlets or brochures [ ]
   - ❑ Members of my family [ ]
   - ❑ Friends or co-workers [ ]
   - ❑ Teachers or lecturers [ ]
   - ❑ Ministers or other spiritual leaders [ ]
   - ❑ Doctors or other medical personnel [ ]
   - ❑ Professional HIV/AIDS educators [ ]
   - ❑ The Internet [ ]

4. How concerned are you about acquiring HIV at work? Tick one.

   - ❑ I am very concerned [ ]
   - ❑ I am moderately concerned [ ]
   - ❑ I am a little concerned [ ]
   - ❑ I am not at all concerned [ ]

5. How concerned are you about acquiring HIV because of your own sexual or drug-using behaviour?

   - ❑ Very concerned [ ]
   - ❑ Moderately concerned [ ]
   - ❑ A little concerned [ ]
   - ❑ Not at all concerned [ ]

6. Do you know or have you ever known someone with HIV infection or AIDS?

   ❑ Yes [ ]
   ❑ I believe so, but I'm not sure [ ]
   ❑ No [ ]

7. If 'yes,' that person is/was (tick one):

   ❑ A sexual partner [ ]
   ❑ An intravenous-drug using partner [ ]
   ❑ A member of my immediate family [ ]
   ❑ Someone in my extended family [ ]
   ❑ A close friend [ ]
   ❑ A friendly acquaintance [ ]
   ❑ Just someone I knew of [ ]

For each question from 8 to 27, record the number of correct responses, incorrect responses, and the number that ticked 'unsure'.

Correct / Incorrect / Unsure

8. This is true in the UK.

9. False.

10. True.

11. False.

12. False. Many people get this wrong because they confuse donating blood with receiving blood.

13. True.

14. False. To date, no one living with someone with HIV or AIDS has become infected from casual contact.

Correct / Incorrect / Unsure

15. True – although literally, the test only implies the *presence* of HIV because it detects the antibody to the virus.

16. False.

17. True.

18. False.

19. True.

20. True. However, the risks involved in woman to woman sex are much less than man to woman, woman to man and man to man.

21. Although theoretically possible, it has never happened and the odds against it are astronomical.

22. True.

23. False. Identity is not the significant factor; behaviour is.

24. False. Although many people with AIDS are living longer and remaining well for longer periods, there is no treatment that can undo the condition of AIDS.

Correct / Incorrect / Unsure

25. False. Although they have been found to contain traces of HIV, the amount is entirely insufficient, under any conditions, to cause HIV transmission.

26. True. There is always a chance, of course, but the truth is that the UK blood supply is now safer than it has ever been.

27. False. You should always choose a doctor or dentist with care, but as long as they are following standard infection control procedures you need not worry about HIV infection.

For questions 28–50, record the number of responses for each level of agreement.

1 2 3 4 5

28. The best answer is 1. The organisation should always find out whether the people it hires are capable of performing the job; 'health' is too vague and too easily the basis for discriminatory behaviour.

29. On the face of it, this seems like a very value free statement of concern; for example, what care worker wouldn't want to know about the health of her or his clients? But in the present context, and in the context of

most discussions about HIV, it usually means 'we have a right to know if our clients are HIV infected'. Therefore, the best answer is 1. 1 2 3 4 5

30. The best answer is 1. There is a difference between being 'entitled' and being curious.

31. The best answer is 1. Legally and ethically, there is no such right; it is based purely on prejudicial attitudes.

32. The best answer is 5. There is no reason why they should not, unless there are documented behaviour problems that specifically relate to the possibility of HIV infection.

33. The best answer is 5. All the available research tells us, again and again, that there is no reason for excluding lesbians and gay men from any sphere of life.

34. The best answer is 5, unless one is using specific invasive procedures. However, most of the time, with proper infection control, even in these situations healthcare professionals pose no risk of HIV infection.

35. The best answer is 1.

36. The best answer is 1.

37. The best answer is 1. No one, no matter who they are or what they have done, deserves HIV infection or AIDS. 1 2 3 4 5

38. The best answer is 1. There is no logical reason why people with HIV or AIDS should not teach or have contact with children.

39. The best answer is 1. The facts indicate that before long nearly everyone will know someone with HIV infection.

40. The best answer is 5. Everybody has the right to determine who does and does not know intimate and potentially damaging facts about their lives.

41. The best answer is 5. Homosexuality is a fact of life, and ought to be treated as such.

42. The best answer is 1. People with HIV or AIDS will not transmit the virus through food preparation.

43. The best answer is 1. Almost everybody working with clients will, as a matter of course, encounter someone with HIV or AIDS.

44. The best answer is 1. Intravenous drug users care about

many things; many, in fact, tend to be very responsible about HIV and other diseases. 1 2 3 4 5

45. This one is very complex; the best answer would probably be 'it depends'. If an HIV infected person intentionally has unprotected intercourse with a lot of people and does not inform them so that she or he can transmit the virus, it is hard not to see such a person as malicious, dangerous and criminal. It does tend to be a 'red flag' statement, however, because HIV intolerant people want to see people with HIV 'put away' and use transmission as a justification. Therefore we will have to say there is no ideal response to this statement.

46. The best answer is 5. Everyone should examine their behaviour in light of HIV.

47. The best answer is 1. There is absolutely no reason for scientists to lie about the facts of HIV/AIDS; if anything, they tend to be conservative in their estimates and conclusions.

48. The best answer is 3. It really depends on the doctor, what procedures she or he is performing, and any possible risk to the patient.

49. The best answer is 1. Such a policy would result in millions of wasted pounds and little impact on the spread of HIV. 1 2 3 4 5

50. The best answer is 1. Though it does challenge some of the assumptions and myths we live by, it does not destroy anything we hold sacred – if anything, it broadens and deepens our values and institutions.

Questionnaire:
Beliefs and Attitudes about Bisexuality and Homosexuality

1. Do you think there are people in the organisation who are homophobic, that is, anti-lesbian, anti-gay or anti-bisexual? (Circle one)

   Yes No Unsure

2. If 'yes', do you think there is homophobia ...
   (Tick all that apply.)

   - ❑ Amongst staff ?
   - ❑ Amongst management?
   - ❑ Amongst residents/clients?
   - ❑ Amongst volunteers?

3. In your opinion, what determines a person's sexual/ emotional orientation?
   (Tick all that apply.)

   - ❑ Heredity
   - ❑ Environment (learning)

- ❑ Brain chemistry or structure
- ❑ Early sexual experiences
- ❑ Personal choice
- ❑ Unknown factors

4. Does your organisation currently have any lesbian, gay, or bisexual ...
   (Circle appropriate response.)

Staff?	Yes	No	Unsure
Managers?	Yes	No	Unsure
Volunteers?	Yes	No	Unsure

5. In your opinion, should lesbian/gay/bisexual staff be 'out of the closet'?

   Yes No

   If 'yes', to whom? (Tick all that apply.)

   - ❑ Other staff
   - ❑ Managers
   - ❑ Residents/Clients
   - ❑ Volunteers
   - ❑ The community in general

If 'no', why not?

____

6. Do you identify yourself as bisexual, gay or lesbian?

   Yes No Unsure

   If 'yes', are you 'out' at work?

   Yes No

   If 'yes', to whom? (Tick all that apply.)

   - ❑ Staff
   - ❑ Managers
   - ❑ Residents/clients
   - ❑ Volunteers
   - ❑ The community in general

Below are a number of statements. Circle the letters which correspond most closely with your honest opinion *about each one.*

Strongly Agree = SA
Agree = A
Neutral = N
Disagree = D
Strongly Disagree = SD

1. Living as a bisexual, lesbian or gay man is a legitimate lifestyle	SA	A	N	D	SD
2. In my experience, lesbians do not hate men, nor do gay men hate women.	SA	A	N	D	SD
3. I would not want to have a bisexual, lesbian or gay friend.	SA	A	N	D	SD

4. I understand why some people prefer to have their emotional, sexual, and social needs met by someone of the same gender.	SA	A	N	D	SD
5. I am sometimes afraid that if I associate with a bisexual, a lesbian or a gay man, that he or she will 'come on' to me sexually.	SA	A	N	D	SD
6. The idea of two women or two men involved in a sexual encounter makes me uncomfortable.	SA	A	N	D	SD
7. I think that people at work spend too much time talking about homophobia and gay/lesbian/bisexual/transgender issues.	SA	A	N	D	SD
8. I am opposed to bisexuals, lesbians and gay men working in jobs where they come into contact with children.	SA	A	N	D	SD
9. Bisexuals, lesbians and gay men should be protected from discrimination.	SA	A	N	D	SD
10. If I associate with someone known as lesbian or gay, I worry that others will think I am also lesbian or gay.	SA	A	N	D	SD
11. It makes me uncomfortable to see people of the same gender display affection in public.	SA	A	N	D	SD

12. The thought of having a bisexual, lesbian or gay son or daughter upsets me.	SA	A	N	D	SD
13. Lesbians and gay men should not have custody of their children.	SA	A	N	D	SD

The following situations are based on actual incidents. In the spaces provided, describe in two or three sentences how you would respond:

Situation One. You are a counsellor in a residential home. You and John, another counsellor, are working together one afternoon. While you are busy with some paperwork, John is talking with a new resident in the next room. Suddenly the resident, obviously upset, appears at your doorway and says, 'I do not want John anywhere near me – he's queer.'

Your response

Situation Two. You are the manager of a centre for young adults with visual impairment. For some weeks now you have been talking to the parents of a blind teenage girl; they are considering letting their daughter come to the centre. On the day they are supposed to come in to sign the necessary paperwork to join the centre, they call you, angry, and ask, 'We were all ready to admit our daughter when we found out that you have homosexuals on your staff – is it true?'

Your response

Situation Three. You are walking past an office in which two colleagues are talking. As you pass the door, you overhear one mention the name of another co-worker, followed by the comment, 'Well, what can you expect of a dyke?'

Your response

Beliefs and Attitudes about Bisexuality and Homosexuality: Scoring

Record number of responses for each in the boxes [ ].

1. Do you think there are people in the organisation who are homophobic, that is, anti-lesbian, anti-gay or anti-bisexual? (Circle one.)

   Yes [ ] No [ ] Unsure [ ]

2. If 'yes' do you think there is homophobia ... (Tick all that apply.)

   ❑ Amongst staff? [ ]
   ❑ Amongst management? [ ]
   ❑ Amongst residents/clients? [ ]
   ❑ Amongst volunteers? [ ]

3. In your opinion, what determines a person's sexual/emotional orientation? (Tick all that apply.)

   ❑ Heredity [ ]
   ❑ Environment (learning) [ ]
   ❑ Brain chemistry or structure [ ]
   ❑ Early sexual experiences [ ]
   ❑ Personal choice [ ]
   ❑ Unknown factors [ ]

4. Does your organisation currently have any lesbian, gay or bisexual ... (Circle appropriate response.)

Staff?	Yes [ ]	No [ ]	Unsure [ ]
Managers?	Yes [ ]	No [ ]	Unsure [ ]
Volunteers?	Yes [ ]	No [ ]	Unsure [ ]

5. In your opinion, should lesbian/gay/bisexual staff be 'out of the closet?'

Yes No Unsure
[ ] [ ] [ ]

If 'yes,' to whom? (Tick all that apply.)

❑ Other staff [ ]
❑ Managers [ ]
❑ Residents/Clients [ ]
❑ Volunteers [ ]
❑ The community in general [ ]

If 'no', why not?

Record comments given.

6. Do you identify yourself as bisexual, gay or lesbian?

Yes No Unsure
[ ] [ ] [ ]

If 'yes', are you 'out' at work?

Yes No
[ ] [ ]

If 'yes', to whom? (Tick all that apply.)

❑ Staff [ ]
❑ Managers [ ]
❑ Residents/Clients [ ]
❑ Volunteers [ ]
❑ The community in general [ ]

Below are a number of statements. Circle the letters which correspond most closely with your honest opinion *about each one.*

Strongly Agree = SA
Agree = A
Neutral = N
Disagree = D
Strongly Disagree = SD

For statements 1–12 record the number of responses for each level of agreement.

	SA	A	N	D	SD
1. The best answer is 'Strongly Agree'.					
2. The best answer is 'Strongly Agree'. The question is based on the myth that people are attracted to members of the same gender because of bad experiences with the opposite gender.					
3. The best answer is 'Strongly Disagree'.					
4. The best answer is 'Strongly Agree'.					
5. The best answer is 'Strongly Disagree'. While it is possible, it should be of no more concern than the possibility that a friend of the opposite gender would make such a move. And if they did, the mature person could handle it with sensitivity.					

	SA	A	N	D	SD
6. The best answer is 'Strongly Disagree', although everyone in society is taught from an early age that such acts are repulsive.					
7. The best answer is 'Strongly Disagree'. Although it is possible that one member of staff may be talking about homophobia a great deal, it is not likely; most people at work see little, if any, discussion.					
8. The best answer is 'Strongly Disagree'. There are a number of reasons why people believe this, but one of the most common is an ungrounded fear that the adult will sexually abuse the child. The overwhelming evidence indicates that heterosexual adults are more likely to sexually abuse children than gay or lesbian adults.					
9. The best answer is 'Strongly Agree'.					
10. The best answer is 'Strongly Disagree', since an individual with self-confidence and high self-esteem would not be concerned.					

	SA	A	N	D	SD
11. The best answer is 'Strongly Disagree'.					
12. The best answer is 'Strongly Disagree', although it would be natural for even a loving, accepting parent to be worried about the homophobia their child will face.					
13. The best answer is 'Strongly Disagree'.					

The following situations are based on actual incidents. In the spaces provided, describe in two or three sentences how you would respond. (Situations One, Two and Three are presented, along with a personal response space.)

It would be impossible to quantify 'correct' or 'most desirable' responses to the three different scenarios, though the answers should be revealing. However, it should be obvious that the 'best' response in each case would be one that was sensitive to the feelings of all parties involved, while at the same time taking a firm stand against homophobia.

8 Taking Action

Steps in Policy Development and Implementation

The process of HIV policy development in most organisations will progress along a series of discernible, tangible steps. A review of those steps, therefore, forms the logical foundation of this book.

1. The organisation has to **decide** that it does indeed recognise the need for a comprehensive policy about HIV and AIDS. On the face of it such a decision seems simple; in reality, there are usually some in the organisation who will advocate for HIV policy, and some who will actively or passively oppose it.

2. The organisation needs to **research** facts about HIV and AIDS, their related policy implications and the legal and scientific premisses upon which good policy rests. Other chapters in this book address most of those topics. There may, however, be specific areas which need to be addressed for particular organisations. This is especially true for organisations in the statutory and independent sector who deal with specific groups, such as working with children, people in prison, homeless people, people with disabilities, mental health problems and learning difficulties.

3. Individuals will need to **survey** and assess the organisation as it is now. They will need to determine which policies in place already speak to aspects of HIV, and evaluate their adequacy. And they will need to find out what staff and clients know and do not know about HIV, and what beliefs and attitudes about HIV dominate the organisation.

4. Members of the organisation will need to take the research and information they have accumulated to date and begin to **plan** for policy development. Draft policy will have to be written. A process for policy implementation will have to be articulated. Staff and client training needs should be determined so that HIV policy, when distributed, is comprehensible to all.

5. The plan will have to be **implemented**. Higher management approval may be required at this point, if they have not already been involved in the planning process.

6. Compliance with implemented HIV policy will have to be **evaluated**. If policy is not being rigorously followed, the policy itself (or aspects of its implementation) will have to be scrutinised and corrected.

Step 1: DECIDING

It always begins with one person.

A company director finds out a family member is HIV positive and decides his business needs to respond. A care attendant works with a client with AIDS and is personally impacted. A counsellor attends an HIV/AIDS workshop and returns to her agency, committed to doing something about HIV. A manager engages in some serious reading about HIV/AIDS and realises that it is only a matter of time before her organisation comes face to face with AIDS.

It has happened hundreds of times: in the end, it always comes down to one person who wants to do something.

For your business or organisation, that one-person policy catalyst might be you, the reader. Assuming that you have already decided that it is important for your organisation to have a comprehensive policy about HIV/AIDS, the next step is a little more difficult. How do you convince the organisation as a whole that it is important to decide?

Decisions for change in most organisations originate from the top and flow down, or at the bottom (or middle) and extend upwards. The two situations are very different, and require different strategic blueprints.

If you are a personnel manager, company director, management committee member or member of the management team you are already in a position to declare the need for HIV/AIDS policy. That does not mean that everybody in your organisation will welcome the prospect, but education and training (which is within your power to put on the agenda and, if necessary, require) can help to convince others that HIV is an important topic, and that comprehensive policy is an appropriate response. But what about the reader who is not in such a position, and who may face opposition? Some advice from others in similar situations might be helpful:

- The process may take time. The organisation may need a period of education to build awareness about the need for policy.

- Do not wait for someone else to take the initiative. Do some research yourself or offer to draft policy.

- If your organisation has a recognised trade union or professional body they may be able to help. 'A number of motions passed at TUC conferences have made it clear that all affiliated unions should adhere to equal opportunities for people with HIV and AIDS. All major trade unions, such as Unison, the GMB and TGWU, have developed comprehensive guidelines and policy on HIV and AIDS. Many smaller unions and professional bodies also have developed specific policy or guidelines. Trade unions and professional bodies with a commitment to equal opportunities should be encouraging employers to adopt policy.

- Find out if other organisations similar to yours in mission and scope have already adopted policy about HIV. If few or none have, you can build an argument for 'enhancing the leadership' of your organisation by beginning to develop HIV policy. If others have implemented policy, you may be able to learn from their experience. You can also build an argument for 'keeping pace' with your competitors or 'being progressive' like other affiliated organisations.

- Investigate laws and guidance which affect your kind of workplace, and whether any are related to HIV. The Disability Discrimination Act (DDA), for example, does have implications for most organisations both as employers and providers of services. A significant number of managers and directors are still unsure about the DDA's potential impact on their organisation. Bring such laws and guidance to your supervisor's attention, and suggest that 'we might need to do something about this' (Chapters 2 and 3 should help you to work out the legal implications in relation to HIV).

- Raise the issue in staff and supervisory meetings. When appropriate, pose dilemmas the organisation may face if it fails to prepare for HIV/AIDS.

- In some organisations, you may be able to suggest inviting speakers to conduct in-service education workshops or circulate articles about HIV/AIDS.

- Analyse sources of support and potential opposition. Sometimes resistance to policy may have nothing to do with HIV/AIDS or its related issues. For example, an organisation in the midst of financial crisis, or experiencing redundancies will be reluctant to take on new challenges that may involve an expenditure of time or money.

- If you do find support from others, you may be able to assemble and activate a planning team. It may not be that everyone in the organisation currently accepts the need for an HIV/AIDS policy, but the process of initiating action, rather than passively waiting for some catalytic event, will itself be educative. It will be hard for top managers, even if they are resistant to the idea of an HIV/AIDS policy, to condemn a planning team's voluntary involvement in a project.

Step 2: RESEARCHING

If an organisation accepts the challenge of HIV/AIDS, policy makers should begin a period of self-education, followed by brainstorming and broad strategic planning. For those settings where management endorsement of HIV policy development is already a given, this will not require much effort.

This step is not nearly as complicated or protracted as it may appear. Management education, for example, might involve nothing more than making a few core reading materials available to management. Discussions of possible impact may take just half an hour in a management meeting. What is essential at this stage is that (1) everybody is brought up to the same basic level of understanding about HIV and HIV related issues, and (2) that individuals engage in some focused dialogue about the future of HIV and the organisation.

Ideas for Researching: Management

Management Self-Education

- Reading materials/videos
- Workshop conducted by local HIV/AIDS expert
- Hearing from people living with HIV or AIDS
- Hearing from representatives or managers of like organisations who have already undergone the policy-making process

Management Brainstorming

- Impact of HIV/AIDS on our organisation five, ten, twenty years from now
- Staffing?

- Work programme?
- Resources?
- Client needs?

Broad Strategic Planning

- What do we need to do to get ready?

Management commitment is certainly desirable, but as already suggested, it is not always the case. The reader who comes from an organisation where management has not committed to a process of HIV policy development is likely to be one of two kinds of staff: first, a manager who has not yet approached a director or executive, and who may expect some resistance when doing so; or second, someone on line staff who has come to believe that policy is important, made a personal commitment to the process, but does not yet know how to proceed or what resistance to expect. Both may, of course, need to carry out some self-education about HIV; a thorough reading of the materials in this book should provide the essentials.

What about strategic planning? At this point, the individuals just mentioned will be more concerned with gaining support for the process within the organisation; a few ideas have already been mentioned. A good point of departure is informal discussion with one's supervisor, asserting the need for HIV policy. Informal education of other staff will also be helpful. The bottom line, however, is that creating the need for change will be up to you; one cannot expect that others will necessarily jump at the opportunity. In such a case, you may need some support and guidance yourself – do not hesitate to seek help and advice from either local or national HIV organisations (ideas of who to contact are given in Appendices 1 and 3).

Whether one begins as an individual hoping for change, or working with a manager and executive staff already committed to change, the next step is to work toward the assembly of a formal or informal team or core group that can carry out research and, later, policy development and implementation. A team approach to HIV/AIDS policy development is highly desirable for several reasons:

- A number of staff, rather than just one person, can learn about HIV and AIDS in the process, making implementation smoother.

- Individuals will be more committed to the success of policy if they helped to create it.

- Soliciting diverse points of view will enable the organisation to create policy that is responsive to real needs – not an abstract document.

- Utilising the energy and resources of a team will help to 'spread the work around' so that no one individual is overwhelmed.

In many small organisations, policy development, as well as many other planning decisions, often follows an informal path. An organisation with a director, five staff and a small management can already function as a 'team' for the purposes of HIV/AIDS policy development. And the process of policy development may indeed be assigned to a single person, providing they enjoy the support of both staff and management.

However, in larger organisations the assembly of a planning team will need to be more deliberate. The team should reflect a range of occupations within the organisation from top to bottom. It should also include key personnel who may be dealing with HIV related concerns and issues. Some of the following grades and occupations could be included within the team:

- Director
- Top manager
- Management representative
- Front-line, direct-service provision staff
- Trade union representative/official

- Personnel manager
- Medical personnel (for example, health and safety representative, company nurse or doctor)
- Staff welfare manager
- Client/customer/service user representative
- For some services, a parent/guardian/partner representative
- Support/maintenance staff representative (e.g. cook, receptionist)

In addition, the team might want to consider adding: an HIV/AIDS expert (someone recommended or from a local or national HIV organisation, health authority or local authority); someone from a high-impact HIV community (gay/bisexual, former intravenous drug user, person with haemophilia); an HIV positive person.

Once the team is assembled, it needs to do its work – develop written recommendations for policy content and its implementation, and shepherd those recommendations through the organisational process of review and adoption. First, however, it needs to carry out more research.

The First Meeting

In the first meeting of the planning team – whether that group is formally constructed or informally gathered – the chair, facilitator or convenor (who is also perhaps the reader) will want to implement four primary objectives, as follows.

(a) Make sure everyone is introduced and has an opportunity to talk about their reasons for being on the team;

(b) Clearly articulate the responsibilities facing the group;

(c) Help the team to make some necessary decisions about research, investigation and surveys to be carried out; and

(d) Conclude the meeting with assignments for the next meeting and an outline of the agendas for coming meetings.

It is suggested that you make available to each team member before the meeting information based on the following material from this book : 'Steps to Comprehensive HIV/ AIDS Policy Development' (following); general background information about HIV and AIDS (sections from Chapter 1 can be used for this purpose); and Chapter 9 which gives suggestions for policy points to be considered in all relevant areas.

At the meeting itself, the facilitator should distribute copies of the agenda; the 'HIV Policy Checklist' and copies of the 'Research Worksheet' (these will be found in the next section, pp. 166–71).

There are a few major decisions to be made in the meeting. First, the team should discuss, and come to some agreement about the current state of HIV policy in the organisation; the 'HIV Policy Checklist' can be usefully employed in that discussion. Second, team members should decide whether to survey the organisation about its HIV related knowledge and attitudes, and if so, which survey instruments to employ. Again, the 'Survey Checklist' and the surveys themselves can aid in making that decision

Finally, a member of the team should be charged with researching one or more of the HIV policy topic areas listed on the agenda (discussed in some detail earlier in this book). Perhaps the easiest way to carry out that task is to have the team member read sections of this book that are related to the policy area, and use the 'Research Worksheet' to summarise notes and suggestions for the next meeting. It should be taken into account that some policy areas are more involved than others to research, and may therefore require more than one team member.

The following section lists the policy areas and outlines the research (including relevant chapters or sections to read in this book) which needs to be carried out by team members.

Policy Areas

Information and training. Researching this area should be fairly straightforward. Chapter 1 has several sections which provide background information about HIV, modes of transmission and so forth. Chapter 9 suggests policy points about how information and training can be disseminated to staff. The person with the task of researching this area should assess the type of information which needs to be given to all or particular groups of staff and make suggestions as to how this can be achieved.

Employment protection. This area is probably the largest area to research because it covers many issues: the extent to which employment law affords protection to people with HIV; victimisation and harassment in the workplace; and conditions of service which may be discriminatory. Relevant reading is: Chapter 2 (HIV in relation to employment law); Chapter 6, which gives examples of the types of problems people have had as a result of HIV discrimination, and the section 'Employment Provisions' in Chapter 9, which suggests policy points that could give equality in employment and conditions of service for people affected by HIV.

Those researching this area need to assess the extent to which the organisation's existing policies and terms and conditions of service cover the above issues.

N.B. There may be considerable overlap with the last section below – Diversity and Equal Opportunities – those researching respective sections should discuss who does what to avoid duplication.

Long-term and intermittent illnesses. Researching this area may be quite involved. The researcher should read Chapter 3 and the relevant section in Chapter 9. The researcher needs to assess how existing company policy deals with long-term or intermittent illness and how it may need to be adapted or changed. The reason this research could be quite involved is that many organisations do not have any specific policies on this area.

Confidentiality. This area should be fairly straightforward to research. It involves reading Chapter 4, the relevant section in Chapter 9 and checking to see what policies the organisation already has on confidentiality.

HIV antibody testing. Again, relatively straightforward to research. It involves reading Chapter 5, the relevant section in Chapter 9 and checking to see if policies already exist to cover testing.

Universal precautions. This book deliberately gives little information about universal precautions in relation to infection control. There is a section in Chapter 1 which gives a general overview. Chapter 9 explains why each organisation must research the issue for itself. The research involved in this policy area may involve little time for small organisations. For larger organisations, especially those involved in health care, it may be quite a large task. The people researching this area may need to contact, for example, the Health and Safety Executive and relevant trade union departments (see 'Useful Information and Addresses' in Appendix 3).

Diversity and equal opportunities. This should be a relatively straightforward area to research, but depends largely on whether or not the organisation already has well developed policies in such areas as race, sexuality and sex. Chapter 6 gives many examples to show how different types of discrimination are interrelated. The chapter also outlines the law in relation to lesbians and gay men. Chapter 9 gives policy points which can be used to address discrimination. The sections 'Employment Provisions' and 'Valuing Diversity and Equal Opportunities for All' are particularly relevant.

Planning Team Agenda – First Meeting

1. Select or confirm chair/convenor/facilitator
2. Team member introductions
   - Who you are
   - Perspective you bring to team
   - Feelings you have about process (e.g. enthusiasm or reservations)

3. Review of team tasks

   - Survey organisation knowledge and attitudes about HIV/AIDS
   - Research policy needs and options (see Checklist, following)
   - Develop draft policy based on research
   - Assess sources of support/resistance within the organisation or larger community
   - Articulate implementation plan, including education and training needs based on survey and assessment
   - Submit draft policy for legal review
   - Offer draft policy and implementation plan to decision makers for action

4. Tasks to be carried out

   - Research

     (a) Knowledge about HIV/AIDS for team (the 'Fact Sheets' pack given to each member of the team before or at the first meeting)

     (b) Policy areas:

     Information and training
     Employment protection
     Long-term and intermittent illnesses
     Confidentiality
     HIV antibody testing
     Universal precautions
     Diversity and equal opportunities

(Members of the team should be assigned to research one or more of each of the policy areas and prepare a brief report for the next team meeting; see Research Worksheet. The materials in this book should be sufficient for most investigation needs in the UK.)

5. Open discussion

6. Confirm assignments and set date for next meeting

Steps to Comprehensive HIV/AIDS Policy Development

1. Deciding

2. Researching

   - Facts about HIV/AIDS

   - Policy implications of facts

3. Surveying/Assessing

   - Existing policies

   - Knowledge/attitudes about HIV/AIDS

   - AIDS and the organisation

   - Beliefs/attitudes about homosexuality

4. Planning

   - Drafting policy

   - Barriers and strategies for overcoming them

   - Education/training plan

5. Implementing

   - Policy legal review

   - Director/management approval

- Communication of new policy
- Training/education:
  - Supervisors
  - Direct service staff
  - Clients
  - Others

6. Evaluating

HIV Policy Checklist

Information and Training

❑ We already have satisfactory policy in this area, and it is being implemented.

❑ We already have effective policy in this area, but it is not being effectively implemented.

❑ We do not have effective policy in this area.

Employment Protection

❑ We already have satisfactory policy in this area, and it is being implemented.

❑ We already have effective policy in this area, but it is not being effectively implemented.

❑ We do not have effective policy in this area.

Long-term and Intermittent Illnesses

❑ We already have satisfactory policy in this area, and it is being implemented.

❑ We already have effective policy in this area, but it is not being effectively implemented.

❑ We do not have effective policy in this area.

Universal Precautions

- ❑ We already have satisfactory policy in this area, and it is being implemented.
- ❑ We already have effective policy in this area, but it is not being effectively implemented.
- ❑ We do not have effective policy in this area.

Confidentiality

- ❑ We already have satisfactory policy in this area, and it is being implemented.
- ❑ We already have effective policy in this area, but it is not being effectively implemented.
- ❑ We do not have effective policy in this area.

HIV Antibody Testing

- ❑ We already have satisfactory policy in this area, and it is being implemented.
- ❑ We already have effective policy in this area, but it is not being effectively implemented.
- ❑ We do not have effective policy in this area.

Diversity and Equal Opportunities

- ❑ We already have satisfactory policy in this area, and it is being implemented.
- ❑ We already have effective policy in this area, but it is not being effectively implemented.
- ❑ We do not have effective policy in this area.

Research Worksheet

Your task is to research one of the outlined HIV/AIDS policy areas, and prepare a report for the next planning team meeting. It is much easier than it may sound; most of what you will need is found somewhere in the information supplied. Basically you only need to answer a few questions.

What are the Facts?

For example, in the area of 'Discrimination', you will want to survey appropriate laws that address (directly or by implication) HIV and discrimination. For 'Infection Control' you will want to review basic principles and procedures. You should be prepared to summarise your findings in an outline, either written or verbal (whichever the planning team has agreed upon).

What do the Facts Imply about Policy?

In your research about fundamental facts you will inevitably draw some conclusions about policy in relation to those facts. For example, you may decide that your organisation needs a specific way of addressing infection control, or that there need to be mechanisms for ensuring HIV confidentiality. Frame your conclusions in brief statements of recommendations.

Notes:

Step 3: SURVEYING/ASSESSING

After the first meeting of the planning team, members will be gathering information in preparation for the next meeting. The primary task for all members of the planning team should be to learn as much as they can – and if the process takes some time, it will be time well spent.

The agenda for the second meeting of the planning team, as follows, moves the team into the third step of surveying and assessing. The main goals of the meeting are to hear reports on policy areas and to initiate surveying/assessing tasks. In addition to sharing what individuals have learned, the team will need to engage in some focused discussion about the organisation as it is. (The facilitator will want to make available the 'Survey Checklist' for team members and distribute copies at the meeting.) Several critical questions enter into that discussion.

1. What policies do we have in place now about HIV; or what policies do we now have that might in some way be related to HIV (e.g. infection control)?
   Are these policies as effective as they could be?

2. What do staff and clients know about HIV?
   Where do they get their information from?
   Is it accurate?

3. What beliefs and attitudes do staff and clients have about human sexuality and sexual behaviour?
   About gay/lesbian/bisexual/transgender people?
   About addiction?
   About other issues that inevitably surface in discussion about HIV?

4. How do staff and clients feel generally about facing HIV/AIDS?

The most effective way to gather such information will be to survey the organisation. Several crucial survey instruments are included in Chapter 7 in the section 'Survey Instruments': one assessing the organisation's 'stage' in relation to HIV/AIDS, another evaluating knowledge and attitudes about HIV, and a third canvassing beliefs and attitudes about homosexuality and bisexuality. They are highly recommended and have been refined from a variety of similar surveys in use over the past ten years. There may also be other surveys that team members have seen that could be added to the list.

By the end of the second meeting the team will have decided: (1) what additional information it is seeking; (2) how that information will be collected (e.g. surveys or interviews); (3) the practical mechanics of data gathering; and (4) who will be responsible for which aspects of data gathering.

Planning Team Agenda – Second Meeting

1. Reports from research

   - Presentations
   - Feedback and discussion

2. Decision making: surveying/assessing

   - What policy is in place?
     Is it adequate?
     Is it being implemented?

   - Whether to survey staff on knowledge and attitudes, and if yes,
     (a) which instrument(s) to use?
     (b) how will the survey be conducted?
     (c) who will photocopy, distribute?

3. Set date of next meeting.

Survey Checklist

❑ HIV and the Organisation
❑ The HIV/AIDS Questionnaire
❑ Beliefs and Attitudes about Bisexuality/Homosexuality
❑ Other Surveys

Step 4: PLANNING

Once the planning team has researched the facts about HIV/AIDS and gathered information about your organisation's knowledge and attitudes, the team can begin developing policy and planning for its implementation. At this point the team will need to accomplish several tasks.

These tasks include:

- Review all of the information the team has assembled.
- Draft policy statements in each of the areas identified.
- Review, discuss, and reach agreement about draft policy statements.
- Develop a plan for policy implementation that includes training of staff and clients.

Many people find the actual process of policy writing unnecessarily intimidating. Even equipped with all the essential facts, they sit down with pen and paper and draw a blank. The truth is that there is nothing mystical about writing policy, and you should not balk at the task, even if you have never done it before. Team members can help each other in the process.

In the third meeting of the planning team, members will take on writing assignments for each of the policy areas, most probably for the area they have already researched. The two planning sheets, 'Draft Policy Statement' and 'Guidelines for Policy Statements', (following) will aid individuals when they sit down to write.

In the fourth meeting, the planning team will share their draft policy statements, discuss them, and hopefully reach a broad consensus on HIV policy. Such may not be the case, so additional meetings may need to be scheduled to allow for more discussion and debate – if it takes a while, that is all right. And in the fifth meeting, or once agreement about the content of policy has been achieved, the group needs to discuss and plan for the implementation of policy.

The agenda, as written, is a good guide to follow in discussing implementation. First, the team should spend some time brainstorming obstacles to, and support for, implementation. What resistance to the new policy do you anticipate? What is that resistance based on? Are there financial considerations, personnel issues, or concerns about reactions from clients or customers? All of these questions should be thoroughly reviewed and written down.

There are several different ways to approach implementation. One could, for example, simply issue new policy and expect that every member of the organisation will follow it without question. Such an expectation might prove unrealistic, unless staff already have advanced and uniform knowledge about HIV and sensitivity to its related issues. Another approach is to issue policy and provide training and education to staff as a follow up after it has been issued. However, this strategy will mean that training and education will be forced to respond to the immediate reactions by staff to policy, rather than follow a careful, step-by-step agenda designed to increase knowledge and sensitivity.

The best approach is to provide for an initial period of training and education so that everyone in the organisation is brought 'up to speed' on baseline HIV facts and issues, and then to release policy, which can be accompanied by more specialised education and training on policy implementation, staff roles and responsibilities in relation to policy, and so on.

In discussing implementation, the following questions may be helpful in general team discussion.

1. How will policy and guidelines in this area be disseminated to staff and/or clients?

2. Is there any education, investigation, or planning that needs to precede or accompany dissemination?

3. Who is responsible for implementation?

4. What consequences are there, if any, for breach of policy and guidelines in this area?

5. Will adherence to the policy and guidelines be considered as a part of regular employee performance review/ appraisal?

6. How will new staff be brought into accord with policy or guidelines in this area?

Planning Team Agenda – Third Meeting

1. Survey results

   - Present survey results

   - Discussion
     (a) What do survey results indicate about potential support for opposition to policy implementation?
     (b) What training/education might be warranted?

2. Policy statements

   - Assignments

3. Set date of next meeting.

Draft Policy Statement

1. Information and training

2. Employment protection

3. Long-term and intermittent illnesses

4. Confidentiality

5. HIV antibody testing

6. Universal precautions

7. Diversity and equal opportunities

Guidelines for Policy Statements

When drafting a policy statement you should attempt to respond to the following questions. If your statement answers all of them clearly and concretely, and is legally and ethically valid, the chances are that the policy will be well written and effective.

- **Why** are we writing policy on this topic?
  What problem or potential problem does this policy attempt to address?
  What is the legal and ethical basis for policy in this area?

- **Who** does this policy pertain to?
  All staff, or just some of them?
  Clients?
  Is someone required to monitor policy compliance?

- **What** concretely does this policy direct individuals or the organisation to do, or not do?

- **When** or under what conditions is this policy operative?
  If the policy statement requires an ongoing activity, according to what schedule is that activity conducted?

- **Consequences** What consequences are incurred, both for individuals and the organisation, if the policy is contravened in some way?

Planning Team Agenda – Fourth Meeting

1. Presentation of draft policy statements

2. Decision making: policy

   - Is there consensus about policy statements, or is additional discussion required?

3. Decision making: implementation

- Group brainstorm
  (a) obstacles to implementation
  (b) support for implementation
  (see brainstorm worksheet, following)

- Discussion
  What can be done to turn obstacles into support?

- Decision
  (a) What is our implementation plan?
  (b) What training/education activities will be required to carry out that plan? (See Training/Education Plan and Staff Education Planning Sheet, following.)
  (c) Who is responsible for carrying out the plans?

4. Set date of next meeting.

Brainstorming Successful Policy Implementation

List the obstacles, support and strategies that you and your team can think of regarding policy implementation (use the following headings to arrange your ideas in columns for comparison purposes).

Obstacles to Policy	*Support for Policy*	*Strategies for Change*
________________	________________	________________
________________	________________	________________
________________	________________	________________
________________	________________	________________
________________	________________	________________
________________	________________	________________
________________	________________	________________
________________	________________	________________
________________	________________	________________
________________	________________	________________
________________	________________	________________

Training / Education Plan

- **Who** is the audience?
  Is there more than one audience, e.g. different groupings of staff?
  Who is responsible for overseeing the training plan, and who will deliver the education?

- **What** is the content?
  Is it the same for everyone, or does it vary according to staff groupings?

- **Why** are we doing training?
  Why did we choose the content as we did – in other words, what are the goals of training?

- **When** will the training take place?
  Before or after new policy is released?
  Does timing matter?

- **How** will the training/education be delivered – videos, written materials, presentations?

- **Cost/evaluation**
  What will be the cost to the organisation, and how will the effectiveness of the training be evaluated?
  Will we conduct pre- and post-tests to measure changes in knowledge and attitudes?

Who	**What**	**Why**	**When**	**How**	**Cost/eval**

Staff Education Planning Sheet

Staff position:	*Has received HIV education covering:*	*Needs HIV education covering:*

Step 5: IMPLEMENTING

Having a plan for implementation of HIV policy is not the same as implementation itself. There are a few details that still need to be taken care of:

1. The policy statements should be assembled into a coherent, overall HIV/AIDS policy package. In other words, someone needs to act as an editor. The outline sheet 'Assembling the Policy Package' should help.

2. The proposed policy may need to be reviewed and approved by competent legal advisers.

3. The policy should be approved by the organisation's management and, if your organisation has one, the board of directors. Since the board and management have already been represented on the planning team, approval should be a formality, but it is a necessary one.

4. The team may want another meeting to review the final policy statement and tighten up plans for implementation and staff training and education.

5. The team should set a time to meet again, perhaps three months after the policy has been released to staff, to review and evaluate the impact and effectiveness of policy.

Planning Team Agenda – Fifth Meeting

1. Final review of policy package
   - Discussion and approval
   - Date to submit to decision makers
2. Review of implementation plan
3. Review of training/education plan
4. Planning team evaluation
5. Set date for policy evaluation meeting

Assembling the Policy Package

The following list outlines the constituent elements of a comprehensive policy package addressing all key aspects of HIV/AIDS. The order is deliberate; different topics build upon each other in a sequential fashion. The reader can use the outline as a framework for the development of organisational policy and as a checklist to make sure all critical topics are addressed.

- [ ] Covering memo from Chair or Executive Director
  The policy statement, when released to staff, should be accompanied by a covering memo which acts as an introduction to the policy and a reinforcement of its importance. The example on the following page is particularly effective.

- [ ] Introduction and Statement of Intent
  The policy should begin with a brief introduction that establishes a rationale for policy and a statement of intent. On the following pages are four examples.

- [ ] Information and training
  (Staff and Clients)

- ❑ Employment protection
  (Discrimination and Conditions of Service)

- ❑ Long-term and intermittent illnesses
  (This section may explains links to other policies on health problems)

- ❑ Confidentiality

- ❑ HIV antibody testing

- ❑ Universal precautions

- ❑ Diversity and equal opportunities

- ❑ Implementation and monitoring plan

Sample Covering Memo

To: All employees of *ANYORG*

From: David Jones, Chair

Re: Attached HIV policy

I need to discuss with you a difficult issue that all of us must come to grips with – HIV and AIDS.

You've probably heard about it on television, read about it, talked about it with friends and co-workers. It seems as though everywhere you turn there are new reports being released, different opinions being expressed.

That makes sense, because AIDS has been designated the number one health problem of the decade. It's affecting men, women, gay people, heterosexuals, black and ethnic minority people, children – and those who care for them. Reliable estimates indicate that nearly 1.5 million people in the world have AIDS and many times that number are carrying the HIV virus.

You've probably also heard that AIDS is blood-borne, which means it cannot be spread through casual contact –

touching, sneezing, coughing, sharing toilets or eating utensils. Because of this, there is no danger to an employee if he or she is working with someone who has HIV or AIDS.

Our primary concerns are ensuring that employees have access to accurate information about AIDS and making certain that, should an employee of *ANYORG* ever contract AIDS, she or he is able to continue working, as long as is advisable, in an environment free of discrimination or mistreatment.

With that in mind, we have adopted the attached policy about AIDS for *ANYORG*. I encourage all of you to read it and, should you have any questions, bring them up with your supervisor. We have arranged employee education seminars to supplement this policy, so that there is ample time to find out about HIV and AIDS and have your concerns addressed.

It's been said before, and it is true: the only weapons we now have to fight the HIV epidemic are education and compassion. I think we can make *ANYORG* a place where people learn what they need to know, and treat each other with dignity and respect.

Sample Statement of Intent

1

It is the philosophy of __________ that all people have the right to be treated with respect and dignity. Because people with HIV and AIDS may encounter problems of discrimination and prejudice in employment and as clients, __________ has taken the responsible position of adopting the following Human Immunodeficiency Virus (HIV) policy and guidelines for all employees. The purpose of the guidelines is to ensure that no one will be denied employment or access to services based on her or his real or perceived HIV antibody status.

The guidelines are intended to be an educational tool and outline the procedures that will be followed as we look at providing counselling, infection control and family support when needed. All service and employment policy pertaining to HIV and AIDS status will be consistent with current legal, epidemiological and medical practice and thought.

We all have a critical role to play in curbing the transmission of HIV, and in assisting those in need of service and support. This is true not only for branches in large cities, but also in small communities. In the past, it may have seemed to many people that HIV was confined to large cities or to certain segments of the population, but it is evident today that AIDS knows no boundaries or borders. Everyone will be affected in some manner by the HIV epidemic.

2

Recognising that HIV/AIDS may pose a significant threat to many clients seeking services from __________, and recognising that there is no foundation for discrimination or separate treatment based on ungrounded fears of casual contact, we affirm the critical role of providing effective policy and education regarding HIV. The education and policy will be intended to (1) reduce the potential for discrimination against people with HIV, and (2) provide education to clients and staff that will help them to reduce their risk of HIV infection.

Since it is currently impossible to determine with perfect accuracy the HIV status of any one individual, HIV related policies operate from the assumption that all staff and residents are currently seropositive for HIV.

3

Public and organisational concerns that participants and staff in our facility should be able to work and attend training without being infected with serious communicable diseases such as AIDS and hepatitis B, require that the management adopt procedures effectively responding to these health concerns while respecting the rights of all participants and staff, including those who are infected.

4

The __________ recognises the employment related rights and concerns of employees who may have HIV infection, as well as the rights of clients, to receive quality services regardless of their health condition. The ________ further recognises its obligation as an employer to provide a safe working environment for all employees and clients, and the public at large. We therefore adopt the following policies and procedures to ensure that those rights are maintained and respected.

Step 6: EVALUATING

Some time after the organisation's HIV/AIDS policy has been implemented (three to six months) the planning team should evaluate the effectiveness of both the policy itself and the policy implementation process. Specifically, the team will want to determine:

- Whether policy is clearly understood by everyone concerned;

- Whether the organisation's staff comprehend and accept the philosophical basis for the policy;

- Whether policy, in all its aspects, is being followed strictly and consistently; and

- Whether any refinements or adjustments in policy need to be made.

If policy implementation seems to be progressing smoothly, the meeting can be informal and an opportunity to celebrate a job well done. If there are problems, a more formal approach might be required. Either way, the planning team should summarise the results of its evaluation and share them with everybody else in the organisation who is affected by the HIV policy.

The agenda, following, provides a framework for the meeting. And by the way, when you have made it this far, congratulations!

Planning Team Agenda – Sixth Meeting

1. Evaluation discussion
   - Is the policy working?
   - Are changess in policy or implementation warranted?
2. Summarise evaluation
   - Who will write a summary and distribute?
3. Celebrate!

9 Key Points for Policy on HIV and AIDS

This chapter may be useful at several different stages of the development of policy described in Chapter 8. For example, it may be useful early on in policy development for ideas about the policy points which could be tailored to suit your own organisation and, later, as a checklist to ensure that all areas of major importance have been included within the organisation's policy.

Section 1 draws on material used in other parts of the book to provide suggestions for points or clauses which can be included in HIV and AIDS policies. Section 2 suggests areas which need to be considered when looking at equal opportunties for all employees and clients. A list of policy points which need to be included for lesbians, gay men and bisexuals is also given.

Many of the policy points in both sections have been extracted directly from previous chapters. Other points derive from problems identified in previous chapters, such as discrimination, and attempt to provide ideas for policy which could address these issues.

The information contained in this chapter is not designed to be a model policy. It is crucial to be aware that policy must be tailored to the needs of each particular organisation. Simply adopting 'ready-made' policy points can easily lead to a document that is too remote or general to reflect the uniqueness or complexity of a specific organisation; the result of such documents is that too often they remain only 'paper policies'.

It is recognised that while some organisations will want to produce a specific policy on HIV and AIDS, some may prefer the approach of incorporating HIV into existing company policies on a number of areas. Another approach is for an organisation to incorporate HIV into specific policies about, for example, long-term health problems and disability. Each approach has its own merits and, what ever the approach, the following points can be adapted for any organisation to adopt.

Section 1: Policies on HIV and AIDS

Introducing Policy

GENERAL POLICY STATEMENT

Attention can be brought to an organisation's policy or position on HIV and AIDS by ensuring that it is included as part of a general policy statement on diversity and equal opportunity. For example:

> This organisation values diversity in the workplace. The organisation is therefore committed to providing equal opportunities to and preventing discrimination against people with disabilities, lesbians and gay men, people affected by HIV and on the grounds of race, colour, nationality, ethnic or national origin, sex, marital status, age and other forms of discrimination. The organisation will take proactive measures to ensure that all policies on equal opportunities are implemented and monitored.

BACKGROUND AND RATIONALE

It is always useful to introduce policy with background information on the subject area and an explanation as to why the organisation has decided to adopt a stance on this issue. An introduction to policy on HIV and AIDS could include:

- an explanation of the words used in the policy, especially, of course, what HIV and AIDS stand for;
- a brief history of the HIV epidemic and the current size of the problem;

- a recognition that discrimination exists against people with HIV in all areas of life, including employment;
- a clear link made with other policies to emphasise that HIV discrimination is often inextricably linked to other forms of discrimination, such as sexuality, race, disability and sex;
- a statement of intent which establishes the rationale for the policy (see Chapter 8 for examples).

The introduction should be short and can refer to other sources, for example guidelines and educational materials, which give a more comprehensive explanation of these areas. Some of the detail in Chapter 1 could be summarised and, if necessary, updated, to provide this type of information.

TRADE UNIONS AND RELEVANT ORGANISATIONS

Before going on to give specific policy points, it should be reiterated that all policy on HIV and AIDS and related areas, and all subsequent revisions, should be discussed and negotiated with relevant trade unions. Negotiation should take place at all stages in the process from initial discussion to eventual implementation and monitoring.

Consulting local authorities, health authorities and relevant HIV independent sector organisations can also be beneficial for the development of policy and initiatives on HIV.

Examples of the type of wording which can be used, modified and adapted for HIV policies are given below under main sub-headings for policy. Many of the phrases used are the same or similar to those which have been used in hundreds of existing HIV policies.

Providing Information and Training

This organisation acknowledges that under Section 2 of the Health and Safety at Work Act, employers have a duty to provide adequate information, instruction and training to their workforce and that this is also part of their common law duty of care.

The organisation notes that the greater the awareness of other staff about HIV related issues, the greater the likelihood of co-operation with company policy and procedures on HIV. The organisation is committed to the following action on information and training.

1. All policy, procedures and guidelines about HIV and AIDS will be clearly communicated to all employees.

2. Information will be available to all staff and (if appropriate) clients of the organisation. The information will document not only the background and facts about the modes of transmission of HIV and AIDS, but also the types of discrimination which people affected have experienced, including sexuality and race discrimination.

3. The information will include telephone numbers and addresses of organisations which can be contacted for more information or advice about HIV and AIDS.

4. All staff with managerial, supervisory and personnel and welfare functions will be given training on HIV and AIDS. (*Or, ideally:* All staff will receive training about HIV and AIDS.)

5. Where training is given, participation and discussion will be encouraged for all involved.

6. All personnel involved in recruitment procedures will have had comprehensive training in equal opportunities, including those relating to HIV.

N.B. *Some organisations have counselling or welfare services for staff. For example, some organisations have 'First Contact Officers' for employees to call in confidence if they have any type of problem they need to talk about. Clearly these staff need to be fully trained in HIV awareness: such people may be the first contact an employee has with another staff member if they are experiencing problems related to their antibody status.*

Employment Provisions

This organisation is committed to effective compliance with all aspects of employment law including: the Employment Protection (Consolidation) Act 1978, the Sex Discrimination Act 1975, the Race Relations Act 1976 and the Disability Discrimination Act 1995.

Moreover, the organisation recognises that people with HIV who are asymptomatic have no specific protection under employment law. The organisation is committed to redressing this imbalance by affording full employment protection to employees or potential employees with HIV.

1. On the basis of medical, legal and ethical considerations, there is no reason to treat a person differently because of their HIV status.

2. No one will be refused employment because they are, or are thought to be, HIV positive or HIV positive and symptomatic.

3. If a successful job applicant is HIV positive and symptomatic, the organisation will seek to make any reasonable adjustments or adaptations necessary in order to employ that person (*see also adaptations and modifications later in this section*).

4. No one will be refused promotion or training because they are, or are thought to be, HIV positive or HIV positive and symptomatic.

5. No one will be dismissed because they are, or are thought to be, HIV positive or because they have a diagnosis of AIDS.

VICTIMISATION AND HARASSMENT

This organisation recognises that people who are HIV positive have experienced a unique form of discrimination because of the prejudice and misunderstanding about HIV.

As an employer, the organisation recognises that it has a duty to prevent harassment and discrimination against people affected by HIV. Therefore:

1. The organisation will aim to provide a safe and supportive environment for people affected by HIV.

2. Training and information will be given in the workplace which aims to eradicate fear about, and combat discrimination against, people with HIV and AIDS (*see above, Providing Information and Training*).

3. Harassment or victimisation of an employee who is, or who is thought to be, HIV positive will be a disciplinary offence.

4. Disciplinary action will be considered for employees who refuse to work with people affected by HIV.

5. Any one victimised, harassed or discriminated against because of their HIV status will have recourse to the grievance procedures.

6. The organisation recognises that people who experience HIV related discrimination may not feel safe to inform senior staff through the normal grievance procedures. The organisation will therefore ensure that all employees are informed about where confidential assistance can be found. (*For example, first contact officer, welfare officer or an outside organisation for advice.*)

TERMS AND CONDITIONS OF SERVICE

1. This organisation is committed to ensuring that any employee affected by HIV, including the partners of people with HIV, should have the same terms and conditions, including employee benefits, as all other employees. To achieve this the organisation will review all **conditions of service**, such as those relating to compassionate,

bereavement and special leave, to ensure that all employees, including same sex and unmarried opposite sex partners, receive equal benefits.

2. The organisation recognises that many of the **informal carers** of people with HIV are same sex partners, friends and relatives. Any employee with a responsibility for caring for a person with HIV related illness will have the right to compassionate, bereavement and special leave. Flexible working conditions will also be considered for the carers of people with HIV.

3. This organisation notes that some insurance companies have tried to exclude people with HIV from cover under company **sickness benefit schemes**. The organisation will therefore review the conditions given under the sickness benefit scheme. If people with HIV are excluded, the organisation will explore alternative arrangements.

4. The organisation notes that some **pension schemes** do not adequately cover death in service and ill-health retirement for people with HIV. The organisation will therefore investigate and monitor the conditions of its own pension scheme to ensure that people with HIV are adequately covered.

The organisation is committed to ensuring that the pension scheme gives survivors' benefits not only to married couples but also to surviving spouse, children, dependents and same sex partners.

CLIENTS AND USERS OF THE ORGANISATION

1. No clients or users of the organisation will be denied a service because of their antibody status.

2. The organisation recognises that, because of discrimination, people with HIV may feel reluctant to use certain services. Therefore, the organisation will aim to provide a

welcoming and non-discriminatory service which positively encourages people with HIV to use the organisation as a resource.

SICKNESS AND ABSENCE

1. Normal rules concerning sickness and absence will continue to operate for people who are HIV positive.

2. If an employee wants to leave work because of illness or if they are genuinely not able to continue to work, this organisation will seek to terminate employment in ways which are most beneficial to the employee: where possible the employee will be offered a package of early retirement on ill-health grounds.

3. Before termination of employment is considered, the organisation will investigate all ways in which adjustments and changes to working conditions can be made in order for an employee to continue employment.

4. Any changes to the job or job description will be made in consultation with the employee concerned and the relevant trade union.

Long-term and Intermittent Illness: Working Arrangements and Adjustment

The following recommendations for policy would be more appropriately placed in a policy which covers long-term and intermittent illnesses and disabilities. It should be made clear in these policies, however, that they do apply equally to people with HIV related illnesses or conditions. Suggestions for points which may be most relevant to people with HIV are:

1. Under Section 6 of the DDA, an employer must take reasonable steps to prevent any physical feature of the premises, or any working arrangements that are made,

from causing a substantial disadvantage to a disabled person. This organisation acknowledges that people with HIV related illnesses or disabilities are covered under this section of the Act. Further, the organisation recognises that being able to continue employment may be crucial for the well-being and self-esteem of a person who has a health problem related to their antibody status.

2. The organisation is committed to complying with the Act and, further, will consider any other possibilities that allow an employee to remain in employment for as long as possible.

3. The organisation will ensure that all [managers, departments, branches etc.] are encouraged to plan in advance to ensure that arrangements can be flexible if any such requests are made.

4. Guidance will be issued which details the types of changes and modifications that can be made to working conditions and arrangements. The guidelines will list the responsibilities that employers have under Section 6 of the DDA and will explain the adaptations and changes which can be made in order to assist a person with HIV related illness to remain in employment. (*The second half of Chapter 3 gives considerable detail about the changes and arrangements that can be made to help people with HIV related illnesses to remain in employment – guidelines could therefore be drafted from this section.*)

Confidentiality

Every organisation, regardless of its types of clients or customers, can adopt the following elements, based on the above principles, into a confidentiality policy.

This organisation will ensure that:

1. All laws relating to confidentiality will be rigorously adhered to.

2. Confidentiality is ensured for all personal and medical information, including an employee's or client's HIV status.

3. Should the fact become known that an employee or user of the organisation has the virus, then strict confidentiality will be maintained.

4. Only those people with a genuine reason to know that a person has HIV will be informed. No one will be informed without the written consent of the person affected by HIV.

5. An employee or client with HIV whose status is known, should be protected from discrimination, and the organisation will aim to ensure this by providing education in the workplace.

6. Deliberate breaches of confidentiality will be considered a disciplinary offence.

HIV Antibody Testing

This organisation recognises that:

- testing employees or potential employees for the HIV antibody cannot give reliable information about an employee's HIV status;

- the mere presence of HIV tells an employer nothing about the individual's capacity to do a particular job;

- the presence of HIV does not give any indication as to whether that person is likely to become ill in the near or even distant future;

- requiring employees to be tested may be open to challenge under employment law;

- being tested for HIV antibodies is a personal and confidential matter for each individual;

- forcing an individual to be tested is a violation of human rights which could have a devastating effect on the individual.

In recognition of these facts the organisation is committed to the following:

1. No employee or potential employee should be forced to take an HIV antibody test against his or her will.

2. Testing will not be used as a screening device for employment or services.

3. If an employee or potential employee has been tested for HIV antibodies, there is no obligation to inform the employer.

Some organisations that deal with clients or residents may need to have policy which incorporates the possibility that the clients or residents may, for example, enquire about or ask if they can be tested for HIV. In such organisations it is important that they have a policy to cover clients and residents as well as employees. The policy here will need to be very specific to the organisation but some general points which can be added are:

4. No one should be tested for the HIV antibody unless true, informed consent has first been given.

5. All individuals have the right to all available information about testing, including the range of opinions about the advantages and disadvantages of testing.

6. Anyone who has decided that they are going to be tested will be advised to ensure that they have the option of pre- and post-test counselling.

7. Anyone requiring to be tested should be encouraged to use GUM clinics where counselling and support services are available.

Universal Precautions

Only a few suggestions for specific policy points are given here. This is because it is essential that each organisation should investigate and check that its procedures relating to health and safety, including standard good procedures for infection control, are up to date, relevant to the current work force and in operation. Appendix 3 gives details about where relevant information can be found.

For most organisations, whether in the private, statutory or independent sector, there is little risk of occupational HIV infection – even in settings where individuals come into contact with blood or other infectious bodily fluids.

In addition, in the vast majority of occupational settings, the precautions which need to be taken against HIV infection are exactly the same as the ordinary health and safety procedures: this is because HIV is harder to transmit than many other infections, such as hepatitis B. Even so, the adoption of policy on HIV is a good time to check that all relevant procedures are in place. Good infection control is wise even in the absence of HIV: it can help to reduce common diseases and infections (colds, flu, and so forth) that tend to spread rapidly through workplaces.

Once procedures have been checked and, if necessary, updated, then the organisation should ensure that:

- all employees are informed of the procedures and of any specific or general responsibilities they may have;
- all employees are given training or information about procedures to follow in the event of accidents at work – including any situation where they may come into contact with blood or other bodily fluids;
- first aiders are trained in and understand all procedures;
- first aiders are given all necessary infection control equipment, such as gloves, aprons, paper towels, bleach, disinfectants.

Section 2: Valuing Diversity and Equal Opportunities for All

If the organisation is committed to valuing the diversity of all its existing and potential staff and clients, then it will want to ensure that it has comprehensive equal opportunities policies (EOPs) which give equal treatment to all staff.

First, all organisations will want to examine existing company policies that relate to equal opportunities in employment and services. Are they sufficiently inclusive? Are all of the groups that experience discrimination covered in the policy?

Second, organisations will want to review their staff and, if appropriate, volunteer make-up, to assess the degree to which it adequately represents the demographic composition of the communities and client base it serves.

Third, organisations will want to commit to the ongoing development of staff competence in relation to diversity issues.

All policy should be planned in consultation with the relevant trade union.

The following advice to employers from the Institute of Personnel and Development (IPD) provides a useful list of policy areas which should be examined in relation to managing diversity. The IPD advises employers to:

- Focus on essential and objective job-related criteria when making employment and training decisions about people.

- Introduce mechanisms to deal with all forms of harassment, bullying and intimidating behaviour. These should indicate that such behaviour will not be tolerated and set out the consequences of breaking the organisation's behaviour code.

- Train widely to encourage an understanding of why valuing people as individuals is important to the organisation.

- Include diversity issues in induction programmes so that all new employees know about the organisation's policies and values.

- Be pro-active in checking for and removing unfair biases in systems, procedures and their applications.

- Encourage employee consultation, involvement, good communication and feedback to make sure the organisation has commitment to diversity management.[1]

Policy Recommendations for Lesbians, Gay Men and Bisexuals

Suggestions are given below for the elements that can be included in policies for lesbians and gay men. They are only summary versions of the issues that need to be covered. The organisation LAGER (Lesbian and Gay Employment Rights) provides information, consultation and training on all aspects of equal opportunities policies for lesbians and gay men (*see Appendix* 3).

1. As with HIV and other forms of discrimination, it is useful to mention lesbians, gay men and bisexuals within a general policy statement.

   It is preferable to mention lesbians, gay men and bisexuals by name as opposed to using the terms 'sexuality' or 'sexual orientation'. The reason for this is that everybody has a sexuality or sexual orientation – including necrophiliacs and paedophiles. It is therefore preferable to name the specific groups that the policy is addressing. If 'sexuality' is to be used in the general policy statement (some argue it is grammatically simpler to do this) then the actual policy should give a definition of what is meant by 'sexuality'.

2. The policy statement should be backed up with a detailed policy for lesbians and gay men.

3. It is important for policy to stress that lesbians and gay men will receive the same employment protection, including protection from dismissal, as any other employees in the organisation.

4. The policy should commit the organisation to challenging and opposing all forms of discrimination against lesbians and gay men.

5. Disciplinary and grievance procedures should state clearly that discrimination against lesbians and gay men will be considered a disciplinary offence.

6. An EOP should state clearly that people have the right to be openly lesbian or gay at work. The policy should also recognise the right of lesbians and gay employees or clients not to have their sexuality disclosed, without their permission, by others in the organisation. In certain circumstances breaches of confidentiality may be considered a disciplinary offence.

7. Many employers do not give the same conditions of service and benefits to lesbians and gay men as they do to heterosexual employees, especially married employees. Many employees in same sex relationships are not given any rights to, for example, compassionate leave, bereavement leave and pension entitlements. The lack of such rights can be extremely distressing when a partner becomes ill or dies.

   A complete and comprehensive review of the existing terms and conditions in an organisation can ensure that conditions of service give the same benefits and perks to same sex relationships as to heterosexual ones.

8. Any conditions relating to maternity, fostering and adoption should be reviewed to ensure that they do not discriminate against lesbians and gay men or anyone who is not in a marital relationship.

9. As an alternative to paternity leave, conditions of service can offer leave for the co-carers of children.

10. There are certain offences that gay men can be charged with which have no direct heterosexual equivalent. The policy should therefore state that personal records or po-

lice records which report criminal offences that have no heterosexual equivalent, shall be ignored.

11. Policy should ensure that no clients are denied services because they are lesbian, gay or bisexual.

12. Training and information should be designed to encourage management and staff to challenge their own discriminatory attitudes and those of others.

13. All policies should include a plan for the implementation and monitoring of the policy.

Appendix 1:
Where Can More Help be Found?

Employers Initiatives: The National AIDS Trust

This section concentrates on the work that the National AIDS Trust (NAT) has done and is continuing to do for employers with a commitment to combating discrimination in employment on the grounds of HIV or AIDS. The reasons for this are twofold. First, because it is important to emphasise that there are already many employers who have successfully adopted or adapted policies to deal with HIV and AIDS in the workplace. The work of the NAT, along with other organisations in the HIV field, has been crucial to this process.

Second, to provide a source of referral for people who are working on HIV and employment policies and strategies: it is recognised by the authors of this book that, although comprehensive in its coverage of HIV and workplace issues, there are some areas for which the reader may need to check that they have the very latest information. The NAT have an *Employers' Initiative* which means that any employer can contact the NAT to discuss their needs in relation to HIV in complete confidence. More detail is given later in this section.

Background

In March 1990 the National AIDS Trust started an employment initiative. The aim was to work out what needed to be done to influence employers to adopt good practice in relation to HIV and AIDS. A result of this initiative was the launch of the 'Companies act!, the HIV/AIDS Business Charter'. The idea was that companies could sign up to the charter provided they were able to demonstrate a commitment to combating discrimination in employment on the grounds of HIV or AIDS. All companies included in the charter signed up to the following wording:

> [This company] is fully committed to the principle of non-discrimination when dealing with an employee or potential employee with HIV. We are also committed to the principle that confidentiality should be strictly adhered to in relation to anyone with HIV or AIDS and that employees or potential employees with AIDS will be treated in exactly the same way as any other member of staff with a comparable disease.
>
> As signatories to 'Companies act!', we demonstrate our commitment through our employment policy on AIDS, in the form of either a separate policy document or specific references within broader employment policies, and by implementing at least one of the following within one year of signing:
>
> Internally:
>
> - providing access to education on HIV/AIDS
> - publicising proven senior management commitment
>
> Externally to play our part in the community by:
>
> - raising the issue of HIV/AIDS in the business community
> - actively and financially supporting Companies act!
> - supporting the work of the National AIDS Trust through sponsorship, donations, or help in kind
> - providing practical assistance to agencies working with HIV/AIDS through help in kind, such as secondments, or funding.

The material sent to the companies gave the following guidelines on the 'Constituents of an equitable AIDS policy'.

> The policy must address both HIV and AIDS separately, and the company's response to each should acknowledge they are separate conditions. HIV and AIDS can be integrated into existing policies, such as those concerning Equal Opportunities, Sickness Leave etc.
>
> - In an integrated policy, mention must be made of HIV and AIDS, to ensure that staff can obtain the information they need on company practice without having to ask specific questions.
> - Any policy must clearly state that discrimination, in any aspect of company activity, against anyone who is HIV positive or who has AIDS will not be tolerated.
> - The policy should state clearly that AIDS will be treated in the same manner as any other progressive or debilitating illness.
> - The policy must contain a clear statement on confidentiality, explaining the way in which confidential information will be treated.
> - The policy must make clear, by outlining or referring to discipline and grievance procedures, what action will be taken if staff breach the terms laid down.
> - The best model policy will cover areas such as opportunities for re-deployment, re-training, flexible working, compassionate leave etc. Where possible these should apply not only to those infected with HIV but also to carers.

The charter was launched in June 1992 with sixteen founder members. By 1996 the number of signatories had risen to fifty and represented a diverse range of organisations. The signatories are listed below:

SIGNATORIES TO THE COMPANIES ACT!
Abbott Mead Vickers/BBDO Ltd
Barclays Bank plc
The Body Shop International plc
Bromley Hospitals NHS Trust
Calibre Films
Cardiff City Council
East Somerset NHS Trust
English National Ballet
Enigma Productions Ltd
General Electric Company plc
Glaxo Holdings plc
HarperCollins Publishers Ltd
Honeywell Control Systems Ltd
IBM United Kingdom Ltd
Newspaper Publishing plc (Independent)
Levi Strauss (UK) Ltd
Lewisham DIREC*Team*
LWT
Marks and Spencer plc
Midland Bank plc
National Association of Citizens Advice Bureaux
National Westminster Bank plc
Nationwide Building Society
Pinderfields Hospitals NHS Trust
London Borough of Richmond upon Thames
NM Rothschild & Sons Ltd
The Royal Ballet
Royal Opera House
Saatchi & Saatchi Advertising
J Sainsbury plc
St David's University College Students' Union
St Helens & Knowsley Health
St Helens & Knowsley Hospitals
WH Smith Ltd
Sotheby's
South Glamorgan County Council
Southend Community Care Services NHS Trust
Sunderland Health Authority
Tayside Regional Council
University of Teesside
Virgin Atlantic Airways Ltd
Woolwich Building Society

Current Services for Employers

In 1997 the NAT launched a new range of services for employers called the 'Employers Initiative'. Any employer can contact NAT's Initiative to discuss their needs around HIV in complete confidence. They will provide advice in response to these initial enquiries. Employers can also access the following range of services for a modest subscription:

- regular news-sheets on the epidemic and the up-to-date information on good practice
- briefing notes on key aspects of HIV and employment
- telephone and postal access to NAT's advice
- help with policy development
- advice on training
- access to events and resources
- access to further consultancy.

A new statement of principles has now also been devised by the NAT which any employer can adopt. The statement is worded to ensure that even the smallest employer is able to give support to the principles. In line with NAT's previous approach, companies do not have to adopt a specific policy on HIV and AIDS providing the key principles are explicitly included in existing company policy and practice. Employers of all sizes and from all sectors are invited to publicly support the Statement of Principles which is reproduced on the following page.

The Statement of Employment Principles for HIV and AIDS

Rationale

HIV and AIDS remain a challenge to employers in the UK. The experiences of many employers have shown that HIV can be managed effectively in the workplace. The National AIDS Trust believes there are key principles to which employers should try to adhere in order to encourage the fair and equitable management of HIV. We believe employers should aim to embrace good practice in four key areas:

The promotion of non-discrimination and consistency

People affected by HIV do not claim the right to any special treatment at work. As indicated by legislation, the management of people with HIV should be consistent with the policy and procedure developed for people affected by other equally serious and potentially progressive medical conditions. Employers should recognise that the fears, prejudices and stigma attached to HIV by some parts of society may prove to be obstacles to consistency. Pre- or post-employment screening for HIV should not be carried out.

Respecting confidentiality

There is a legal requirement that employers safeguard the confidentiality of their employees' personal and medical information. When HIV status is known, the methods devised for the management of that information at work should avoid any unnecessary and damaging disclosures.

The creation of an understanding and supportive environment

Wider awareness of HIV can lead to greater understanding and support for the people it affects. Employers should inform their employees about HIV, thus also ensuring their continued health and safety. By making positive responses to HIV, employers can also contribute to a growing climate of acceptance of HIV and those it affects in the wider community.

Ensuring an informed response to the needs of people affected by HIV and AIDS

Employers should recognise that asymptomatic HIV infection presents its own challenges and may be best approached as an equal opportunities issue, which highlights the dangers of prejudice and discrimination. Illness or disability arising from HIV infection requires management in line with other progressive medical conditions and in accordance with the law. Policy and practice should be developed to meet both of these challenges.

To contact the NAT for more information see Appendix 3.

The material in this section was taken from information supplied by Julian Hussey on behalf of the NAT and from the report, 'Employment and AIDS: A review of the Companies act! business charter on HIV and AIDS', by Julian Hussey. August 1996. Produced by the NAT.

Appendix 2: The UK Declaration of the Rights of People with HIV and AIDS

One of the ways in which an organisation can show commitment to ending discrimination against people affected by HIV is to give its support to the following Declaration. The Declaration was produced by the UK Forum on HIV and Human Rights and was first launched in 1992. Since that time many individuals, groups and organisations have signed up to the Declaration.

The Declaration is a synthesis of all the rights which the UK Government has agreed, in international treaties and covenants, to uphold for all its citizens, together with proposals for implementation of those rights with reference to people with HIV and AIDS.

Any individual, group or organisation wanting to support the declaration can do so by contacting the UK Forum on HIV and Human Rights c/o Immunity (see Appendix 3). The Declaration is printed in full below.

The UK Declaration of the Rights of People with HIV and AIDS

Preface

This declaration is made by people with HIV and AIDS and by organisations dedicated to their welfare. The Declaration lists rights which all citizens of the United Kingdom, including people with HIV and AIDS, enjoy under international law; the Declaration then prescribes measures and recommends practices which the writers of the Declaration believe are the minimum necessary to ensure that these rights are respected and protected within the United Kingdom.

The Declaration

All citizens of the United Kingdom, including people with HIV and AIDS, are accorded the following rights under international law:

- the right to liberty and security of person
- the right to privacy
- the right to freedom of movement
- the right to work
- the right to housing, food, social security, medical assistance and welfare
- the right to freedom from inhumane or degrading treatment
- the right to equal protection of the law and protection from discrimination
- the right to marry
- the right to found a family
- the right to education

These rights exist in international treaties[1] which the United Kingdom Government has agreed to uphold. But these rights, as they apply to United Kingdom citizens with HIV and AIDS, have not been adequately respected or protected. We therefore make a public Declaration of the Rights of People with HIV and AIDS and of our commitment to ensuring that they are upheld.

Liberty and Security

People with HIV and AIDS have the right to liberty and security of person, and in respect of this right we believe that:

1. no person should be subjected to forcible detention, isolation, or segregation from society purely on the grounds of their having HIV, or having AIDS or an AIDS-related condition;

2. no prisoner should be segregated from other prisoners purely on the grounds of their having HIV, or having AIDS or an AIDS-related condition.[2]

We affirm and hold, in agreement with the World Health Organisation, that 'persons suspected or known to be HIV-infected should remain integrated with society ...'

Privacy

People with HIV and AIDS have the right to privacy, and in respect of this right, we believe that:

3. information about the HIV status of any person should be kept confidential to that person and their appointed health and social carers (except where anonymous information is given to a public body for the purpose of studying the epidemiology of HIV);

4. information should not be disclosed to a third party about a person's HIV status without that person's consent;

5. in accordance with a judgement of the European Court of Human Rights, the right to privacy includes the right 'to establish and develop relationships with other human beings, especially in the emotional sphere, for the development and fulfilment of one's own personality'.[3]

Freedom of Movement

People with HIV and AIDS have the right to freedom of movement, and in respect of this right we believe that:

6. no restrictions should be placed on the free movement of individuals within and between States purely on the grounds of their having HIV, or having AIDS or an AIDS-related condition.

We affirm and hold, in agreement with the Committee of Ministers of the Council of Europe, that 'in the light of present knowledge, discriminatory measures such as control at borders ... should not be introduced as they are not justified either scientifically or ethically'.[4]

Work

People with HIV and AIDS have the right to work, and in respect of this right we believe that:

7. no person should be barred from employment or dismissed from employment purely on the grounds of their having HIV, or having AIDS or an AIDS-related condition;

8. employers should ensure that their terms and conditions of employment are such as to enable people with HIV, AIDS or an AIDS-related condition to continue in their employment, and to do so in a healthy and safe working environment;

9. employers or their agents should not perform tests to detect the HIV status of current or prospective employees;

10. in respect of the right to work, the right to privacy, and the right to protection from discrimination, there should be no obligation or requirement upon an individual to disclose to an employer their own HIV status, or the HIV status of another person.

Housing, Food, Social Security, Medical Assistance and Welfare

All persons, including those with HIV and AIDS, have the right to housing, food, social security, medical assistance and welfare.

In respect of the right to housing, food and social security, we note that Article 11 of the International Covenant on Economic, Social and Cultural Rights states:

> The parties to the present covenant recognise the right of everyone to an adequate standard of living for himself and his family, including adequate food, clothing and housing ...

In respect of these rights, we believe that individuals with HIV and AIDS, and their dependants, who are in social or housing need, should be offered:

11. the prompt provision of housing which is beneficial to their physical and mental well-being;

12. the provision of adequate means, through direct financial assistance and provision by appropriate social care agencies, to maintain a reasonable standard of living and especially an appropriate diet.

In respect of the right to medical assistance and welfare, we believe that people with HIV, AIDS or an AIDS-related condition should have:

13. full access to available medical treatment, including complementary and experimental therapies, without charge to the recipient;

14. access to blood products of the highest quality, for those dependent on them;

15. free access to a data-base providing information about therapeutic research in relation to HIV infection, AIDS and associated conditions;

16. access to the provision by statutory and voluntary agencies of social care by appropriately trained workers;

17. for those who have problems with illegal substances, access to a full range of services (including maintenance therapy) that is appropriate to their needs;

18. care unprejudiced by the agreement or refusal to participate in research trials.

In relation to social and medical care, we believe that people with HIV and AIDS should:

19. be fully involved in a working partnership with medical, health and social care workers and researchers to develop policies and practices which meet their medical, health and social care needs.

In relation to medical care, we believe that people with HIV and AIDS should:

20. be able to refuse treatment or restrict their treatment to palliative care.

In respect of the right to medical assistance, and of the duty of Governments to protect the health of citizens, we urge the United Kingdom Government to allocate a proper proportion of available resources towards therapeutic research into HIV infection and conditions associated with AIDS.

Equal Protection of the Law and Protection from Discrimination

People with HIV and AIDS have the right to equal protection of the law and protection from discrimination. We note the statement of the World Health Organisation that:

> The avoidance of discrimination against persons known or suspected to be HIV-infected is important for AIDS

prevention and control: failure to prevent such discrimination may endanger public health.[5]

In respect of the right to protection from discrimination we believe that:

21. measures should be taken to protect people with HIV and AIDS from discrimination in the areas of employment, housing, education, faith, legal services, child care and the provision of medical, social and welfare services, and from arbitrary and commercially unjustified discrimination by private insurance companies;

22. there should be other appropriate provision to protect people with HIV and AIDS, and their dependants, from social disadvantage arising from commercially justified discrimination by private insurance companies.

We note that the World Summit of Ministers of Health on Programmes for AIDS Prevention (hosted and attended by the UK Government) emphasised in the London Declaration on AIDS Prevention (1988) 'the need in AIDS prevention programmes to protect human rights and human dignity' and undertook to 'forge, through information and education and social leadership, a spirit of social tolerance'. In pursuit of this, we believe that:

23. there should be public education whose specific objective is the elimination of discrimination against people with HIV and AIDS.

In support of the above we note that Article 26 of the International Covenant on Civil and Political Rights (which is binding on the United Kingdom Government) states:

> All persons are equal before the law and are entitled without any discrimination to the equal protection of the law. In this respect the law shall prohibit any discrimination and guarantee to all persons equal and effective protection against discrimination on any ground such as race, colour,

sex, language, religion, political or other opinion, national or social origin, property, birth or other status.

We submit that HIV status and HIV-related disability fall within the 'other status' covered by this prohibition of discrimination.

To Marry and to Found a Family

People with HIV and AIDS have the right to marry and the right to found a family, and in respect of these rights we believe that:

24. full and appropriate counselling and information, which respects their right to parent children, and the right of women with HIV to bear children, should be made available to those people with HIV and AIDS who wish to exercise this right.[6]

Education

People with HIV and AIDS have the right to education, and in respect of this right:

25. education should not be impaired by restrictions on social interaction placed on people with HIV and AIDS in educational settings.

We believe that these measures are necessary to ensure that the rights of people with HIV and AIDS, and of others disadvantaged as a result of disability or medical condition, are protected in a society which respects the value and dignity of its members.

Appendix 3: Useful Information and Addresses

Specialist Advice and Consultancy

The National AIDS Trust (NAT)

See Appendix 1 for detailed information about the NAT. Also available from the NAT is a list of trainers and training organisations.

Contact Julian Hussey at:
The National AIDS Trust, New City Cloisters,
188/196 Old Street, London EC1V 9FR

Employers' Initiative. Direct Line Tel: 01225 404 964
0171 216 0111
email: info@nat.org.uk
Internet: http://www.nat.org.uk/nat/

The Employment Medical Advisory Service

See the phone book under EMAS or Health and Safety Executive. Offers free advice on all occupational health matters, including AIDS/HIV.

LAGER (Lesbian and Gay Employment Rights)

Provides advice to employers on all aspects of a planned approach to HIV/AIDS issues. Also provides publications, consultancy and training on equal opportunties for lesbians and gay men.

Contact: LAGER
Unit 1G, Leroy House, 436 Essex Road, London N1 3QP
Tel: 0171 704 6066
Fax: 0171 704 6067

Terrence Higgins Trust (THT)

Offers information, help and advice on AIDS/HIV infection and prevention and training courses for managers and staff.

Contact: Terrence Higgins Trust (THT)
52–54 Grays Inn Road, London WC1X 8JU
0171 831 0330 (administration)
0171 242 1010 (helpline: noon–10 p.m. daily)
0171 405 2381 (legal line: Mon. and Wed.)

Immunity Legal Centre

Offers free specialist legal advice to anyone affected by HIV or an AIDS related condition. Although the service is primarily aimed at individuals, training and talks are given to organisations about HIV and the law. The UK Forum on HIV and AIDS can also be contacted c/o Immunity.

Contact: Immunity
1st Floor, 32–38 Osnaburgh Street, London NW1 3ND
Tel: 0171 388 6776
Fax: 0171 388 6371

HEALTH PROMOTION AND HEALTH EDUCATION

Advice and consultancy are available from most local and health authority health promotion units and voluntary groups.

The four national health promotion agencies, which are responsible for health education are:

Health Education Authority
Hamilton House, Mabledon Place, London WC1H 9TX
Tel: 0171 383 3833

Health Education Board for Scotland
Woodburn House, Canaan Lane, Edinburgh EH10 4SG
Tel: 0131 447 8044

The Health Promotion Agency for Northern Ireland
18 Ormeau Avenue, Belfast BT2 8HS
Tel: 0123 231 1611

Health Promotion Wales
Ffynnon-Las, Ty Glas Avenue, Llanishen, Cardiff CF2 1EB
Tel: 0122 275 2222

Disability and HIV Issues

Disability organisations which have taken on work related to HIV and employment include:

The Access to Work Scheme

Contact local Job Centres for information via the Placement, Assessment and Counselling (PAC) Teams.

OUTSET

An organisation dealing primarily with IT training for people with disabilities, including people with HIV/AIDS. The IT training includes placements with employers.

Contact: OUTSET
Drake House, 18 Creekside, London SE8 3DZ
Tel: 0181 692 7141

RNIB (Royal National Institute for the Blind)

For people with any type of visual disability, whatever the cause, services are available for helping in employment related matters.

Contact: The Employment Unit
RNIB, 224 Great Portland Street, London W1N 6AA
Tel: 0171 388 1266

Useful Publications and Resources

The National AIDS Manual

The most comprehensive and regularly updated source of information about all HIV related topics can be found in the *National Aids Manual* (*NAM*). The manual comprises a directory of HIV related contacts and addresses, a volume about treatment in relation to HIV and a volume about topics related to HIV. It is recommended for any organisation that wants to keep up to date with HIV related issues. It is especially recommended for organisations that deal with specialist issues.

Examples of the specialist areas covered by the manual are: epidemiology and research, HIV transmission, HIV prevention methods, safer sex, drug use, HIV testing, making a 'living will', caring for someone with AIDS, housing, immigration, the law and HIV, confidentiality, European law, employment, haemophilia, sex workers, children and families, prisons.

There is an annual subscription and all information is updated at least yearly. A database is also available on subsciption that gives information on all HIV and HIV related services.

Contact:
The National AIDS Manual, NAM Publications,
52 The Eurolink Centre, 49 Effra Road, London SW2 1BZ
Tel: 0171 627 3200
Fax: 0171 627 3101
e-mail: admin@nam.org.uk

Glaxo Wellcome Positive Action

Have produced a Positive Action Employee HIV/AIDS Awareness Programme which consists of information leaflets, an award-winning video, a presentation pack and briefing for managers on how to conduct sessions. In 1996/97 the programme is being instigated for all of its 55,000 global workforce. The pack has been designed primarily for internal use but can be used by other companies either as a whole, or as a resource for developing their own programmes.

For further information contact:
Ben Plumley, Positive Action Co-ordinator,
Glaxo Wellcome plc, Glaxo Wellcome House,
Berkeley Avenue, Greenford, Middlesex UB6 0NN
Tel: 0181 966 8371
Fax: 0181 966 8827

The Industrial Society

Produces the HIV and AIDS Information pack. It contains copies of the actual policies that a range of organisations have adpopted on HIV and AIDS and costs £50.00.

The Industrial Society also produce a useful book called *The Disability Discrimination Act 1995: Putting the Law into Practice* by Jo Gardiner. The book gives general and detailed information about the Act and how it applies to employers and service providers.
The pack and book are available from:
The Information Service, Industrial Society
48 Bryanston Square, London W1H 7LN
Tel: 0171 262 2401

OXAIDS

Produces the 'OXAIDS Business Pack – HIV and AIDS Awareness in the Workplace' by Jane Hatfield (ed.). Information on HIV and the workplace covering first aid, policy implications, overseas travel and AIDS awareness training.

Available from:
OXAIDS, 43 Pembroke Street, Oxford OX1 1BP

EASAH
The Employer's Advisory Service on AIDS and HIV

Publications include: 'The AIDS Leader' which looks at

corporate responses, especially in relation to managing people with compromised immunity and 'Working with AIDS: a guide for businesses and business people'.
Also provides consultancy services.

Contact:
EASAH, PO Box HP 346, Leeds LS6 1UL
Tel: 0113 294 1212
Fax: 0113 294 1313

Health Education Authority (HEA)

Produces a range of publications on HIV and AIDS. 'HIV and AIDS at Work: How to set up an HIV/AIDS policy' is aimed at employers, trade unions and health professionals. Some HEA publications are aimed at specific occupations, for example, seafarers. See 'Health Promotion' above for address.

Health and Safety / First Aid at Work

The Health and Safety Executive and the Department of Health AIDS Unit provide written guidelines for various occupations, especially in the National Health Service. Advice on first aid at work is available from the British Red Cross Society, the St John's Ambulance Brigade or, in Scotland, the St Andrew's Association.

Government Guidelines for Employers

'AIDS and Work: the facts employees should know'
(Dept of Employment), a leaflet endorsed by TUC, NAT, ACAS, CBI, HEA, IPD and HSE.

'AIDS and the Workplace: a guide for employers '
(DoE and the H&S Executive).

These publications should be available at local Health and Safety Executive offices.

Employment Abroad

The UK NGO AIDS Consortium

A networking organisation for charities sending employees to developing countries. The consortium has published two booklets called 'HIV/AIDS & Overseas Employment'. One booklet is for employers, the other for employees. The booklets are published and available from the Health Education Authority (HEA).

For more information about working abroad contact:
Sue Lucas
UK NGO AIDS Consortium for the Third World
Fenner Brockway House,
37–39 Great Guildford Street, London SE1 0ES
Tel: 0171 401 8231

The Confederation of British Industries

Produce a booklet called 'AIDS & Overseas Business Travel' available from:
Centre Point, New Oxford Street, London WC1 1DU

Flexible Working Arrangements

New Ways to Work

An organisation which produces information on flexible working hours, job sharing, working from home and voluntary reduced hours.

Contact:
New Ways to Work,
309 Upper Street, London N1 2TY
Tel: 0171 226 4026

Statistics on HIV and AIDS

Every three months the HIV, STD Division of the Communicable Diseases Surveillance Centre (CDSC) publish comprehensive statistics about HIV and AIDS.

Contact: Public Health Laboratory Service (PHLS),
Communicable Disease Surveillance AIDS Centre
61 Collindale Avenue, London NW9 5EQ
Tel: 0181 200 6868
Fax: 0181 200 7868
Internet: http://www.open.gov.uk/cdsc/cdschome.htm.

Trade Unions and Professional Associations

The Trades Union Congress

Offers a training pack and a joint statement on AIDS (with the CBI and ACAS).

Available from: TUC Publications
Congress House, Great Russell Street, London WC1B 3LS

Some unions have issued their own guidelines and codes of good practice. UNISON, for example, has produced several comprehensive publications on HIV and AIDS. Many unions, however, have produced guidelines which address issues specifically to do with the industry or sectors they represent: some of the guidelines, therefore, do not necessarily carry information on the broader issues on HIV and AIDS or about safer sex.

The Labour Research Department

Publishes a useful booklet for trade unionists, 'HIV, AIDS and the workplace: a trade unionists guide'.

Contact:
The Labour Research Department
78 Blackfriars Road, London SE1 8HF

Help for Individuals

There are many hundreds of organisations which give advice and information about HIV and AIDS to individuals. Some local groups are listed in the community section of the phone book.

A national information service where advice can be sought is:

National AIDS Helpline

A free 24-hour confidential service with helpful, sympathetic staff who can offer information, help and advice on questions relating to HIV and AIDS.
Tel: 0800 567123

Help is also available in the following languages:

Welsh: 0800 371131 (10 a.m. – 2 p.m. daily)

Bengali: 0800 371132 (6 p.m. – 10 p.m. Tuesday)

Punjabi: 0800 371133 (6 p.m. – 10 p.m. Wednesday)

Gujarati: 0800 371134 (6 p.m. – 10 p.m. Wednesday)

Urdu: 0800 371135 (6 p.m. – 10 p.m. Wednesday)

Hindi: 0800 371136 (6 p.m. – 10 p.m. Wednesday)

Cantonese: 0800 282446 (6 p.m. – 10 p.m. Monday)

Arabic: 0800 282447 (6 p.m. – 10 p.m. Thursday)

At other times there is a recorded message on the above lines.

Notes

Notes to Chapter 1

1. In the section 'Researching' in Chapter 8 it is suggested that the information in this chapter could be used as background information for a planning team/policy makers.
2. The information presented on risk reduction is only basic material. A wealth of information is already available about risk reduction, especially in relation to safer sex and drug use. For example, the first HIV organisation in the country, the Terrence Higgins Trust (see Appendix 3) carries out a variety of initiatives, including publications, to promote the adoption of safer sex. In addition, many health promotion units within health authorities produce information on safer sex and risk reduction.
3. Every three months HIV, STD Division of the Communicable Diseases Surveillance Centre (CDSC) (see Appendix 3) publish a comprehensive list of tables which give the number and characteristics of people with HIV and AIDS. All the information in this section is from or deduced from their AIDS/HIV Quarterly Surveillance Tables or reports which are published by the Public Health Laboratory Service AIDS Centre (HIV, STD Division, Communicable Diseases Surveillance Centre) and the Scottish Centre for Infection & Environmental Health. Readers can therefore update figures by contacting the CDSC.
4. From Table 1 of the 'Communicable Diseases Report'. Volume 7, No. 4. January 1997. Produced by CDSC. Ibid.
5. 'AIDS/HIV Quarterly Surveillance Tables', op. cit. No. 32: Data to end June 1996. Table 10.
6. CDSC figures do not report cases of HIV being transmitted by lesbian sex. It cannot be assumed, however, that

all of the women, including those who acquired HIV by drug use, would define themselves as heterosexual.

7. These percentages were worked out from the total number of cases where transmission was known from Table 2 of the 'Communicable Disease Report' Volume 6, No. 42. October 1996. Published by CDSC, op. cit.
8. Ibid.
9. Op. cit. No. 32: Data to end June 1996. Table 26 gives the cumulative number of AIDS cases reported by exposure category and ethnicity. The percentage is derived from a base number of 10,483 cases where ethnicity was recorded and 1801 people who were defined as Black, Asian, Oriental, mixed race or from a category other than white; of these 1801 people, 611 were women and 504 people acquired the virus through male to male sex.

Notes to Chapter 2

1. Department of Employment and the Health and Safety Executive 'AIDS and the Workplace: A guide for Employers' (1989). Page 4.
2. Ibid. Page 6.
3. General Medical Council (GMC), 'HIV and AIDS: the ethical considerations: Guidance from the General Medical Council' (1995). Page 4.

Notes to Chapter 3

1. The Minister for Disabled People, 'A brief guide to the Disability Discrimination Act', DL40. (1996).
2. Department of Employment and the Health and Safety Executive, 'AIDS and the Workplace: A guide for Employers', (1989). Page 2.

Notes to Chapter 4

1. Christopher Southam and Gillian Howard 'AIDS & Employment Law'. Published by Financial Training. Page 183.

2. General Medical Council (GMC) 'HIV and AIDS: the ethical considerations: Guidance from the General Medical Council' (1995). Page 7.

Notes to Chapter 5

1. 'HIV, AIDS and the Workplace: A trade union guide', published by the Labour Research Department, December 1995.
2. Ibid pages 23–24.
3. 'HIV and AIDS: the ethical considerations: Guidance from the General Medical Council'. Page 4.

Notes to Chapter 6

1. Based on information from the AIDS/HIV Quarterly surveillance Tables No. 32: Data to end June 1996. Published by the Public Health Laboratory Service AIDS Centre (HIV, STD Division, Communicable Diseases Surveillance Centre) and the Scottish Centre for Infection & Environmental Health. Table 26, for example, gives the cumulative number of AIDS cases reported by exposure category and ethnicity. Figures are not reported about the ethnicity of people generally with HIV infection.
2. 'Unequal Opportunities: CAB evidence on discrimination in employment', published by NACAB, 1994. Page 44.
3. Ibid.
4. 'Immunity Annual Report 1994–95', published by Immunity. Page 10.
5. Phil Greasley, 'HIV & AIDS Continued Employment Guidelines for Employers', published by LAGER (1992).
6. Jonathan Glasson 'Luxury or Necessity? HIV and Human rights: A Policy Overview', published by the UK Forum on HIV & Human Rights, 1995. Page 11.
7. 'Women like us: Positively Women's survey on the needs and experiences of HIV positive women', published by Positively Women, 1994.
8. Op. cit. Page 20.

9. Op. cit. Page 5.
10. Op. cit. Page 22.
11. Dawn Snape, Katrina Thompson and Mark Chetwynd, 'Discrimination against Lesbians and Gay Men: A study of the nature and extent of discrimination against homosexual men and women in Britain today', published by Social and Community Planning Research (SCPR), (1995). Page vii.
12. Ibid. Page 30.
13. Ibid.
14. 'Managing Diversity', press information. Institute of Personnel and Development, December 1996. Page 2.
15. Ibid. Page 3. Other survey-based research which documents discrimination against lesbians and gay men can be found in the 'Less equal than others – a survey of lesbians and gay men at work'. Published by Stonewall, 1993. Also, see 'Gay men at work: a survey of gay men in employment in London' by Phil Greasley. Published by LAGER, 1986.
16. LAGER casework example reported in the LAGER Annual Report 1994.
17. Example taken from a LAGER press release, October 1996. Contact LAGER for more information about cases in relation to lesbians and gay men (address and phone number in Appendix 3).

Note to Chapter 7

1. Adapted from 'Responding to HIV in Minnesota's Workplaces: A Guide for Chief Executives and Their Managers', (May 1992). Minnesota AIDS Funding Consortium, 1120 Norwest Center, St Paul, MN 55101. (612) 224–5463.

Notes to Chapter 9

1. 'Managing Diversity', an IPD position paper (1996). The paper is available to both IPD members and non members free on request. An A4 sae should be sent to the Institute of Personnel and Development, Policy Group, IPD House, Camp Road, London SW19 4UX.

Notes to Appendices

1. The relevant treaties, which the UK Government has agreed to uphold, are the International Covenant on Civil and Political Rights, the International Covenant on Economic, Social and Cultural Rights (1976), the European Convention on Human Rights (1953) and the European Social Charter (1965).
2. 'Social Aspects of AIDS Prevention and Control Programmes' (World Health Organisation, Geneva, 1987).
3. *Dudgeon* v. *United Kingdom*, Judgement of the European Court of Human Rights (1981) 4 EHRR 149.
4. Appendix to Recommendation No.R (87) 25, para 2.2.2.
5. 'Social Aspects of AIDS Prevention and Control Programmes' (World Health Organisation, Geneva, 1987).
6. Where a woman with HIV or AIDS chooses to have a child, it should be the right of both the woman and the child that the mother be given full support and that all possible procedures be adopted to minimise the risk of HIV transmission from mother to child before, during and after birth.

Index

Index by Judith Lavender